Building Cancer Resistance

DAVID HAZARD

HARVEST HOUSE PUBLISHERS
Eugene, Oregon 97402

Unless otherwise indicated, all Scripture quotations are taken from the King James Version of the Bible.

Cover by Left Coast Design, Portland, Oregon

Advisory

Readers are advised to consult with their physician or other medical practitioner before implementing the suggestions that follow. This book isn't intended to take the place of sound medical advice or to treat specific maladies.

Neither the author nor the publisher assumes any liability for possible adverse consequences as a result of the information contained herein.

BUILDING CANCER RESISTANCE
Copyright © 2001 by David Hazard
Published by Harvest House Publishers
Eugene, Oregon 97402

Library of Congress Cataloging-in-Publication Data
Hazard, David.
    Building cancer resistance   /   David Hazard.
      p. cm.
    ISBN 0-7369-0480-8

Printed in the United States of America.

01 02 03 04 05 06 07 / BP-VS / 10 9 8 7 6 5 4 3 2 1

Contents

Special thanks to
Brian D.F. Richmond, M.P.H.,
for his review and advice in the
development of this book.

Healthy Body, Healthy Soul

"There is new ammunition in the war against cancer!" announces the front headline on a major weekly newsmagazine. Then, referring to the pile of yellow drug capsules pictured on its cover, it declares: "*These* are the bullets."

Inside, though, we learn that this new "miracle" drug "does not help everyone." And it has some very unpleasant side effects. *And,* though this drug has sent certain cancers into remission, it does not *cure* the cancer. In time, cancer may come back.

We are all eagerly awaiting the day when medical and pharmaceutical researchers discover the "magic bullet" that will wipe out cancer. And though more drugs are being tested all the time, a sure-cure drug still eludes us.

*In the meantime…*what can we do if cancer has struck close to us and we're concerned about prevention? What can we do if we have cancer *now* and want to build our resistance and increase our chances of recovering full health?

More and more people are turning to natural medicines—to remedies and simple therapies that have been used, sometimes for centuries—for the prevention and treatment of the various forms of cancer. They are turning back to a simple and ancient approach to health. Namely, that the body is made to repair itself and overcome disease *if* we learn how to keep the various aspects of our being—body, mind, and spirit—in a healthy balance. Today, there is a new and marked cooperation between traditional healthcare practitioners, their patients, and practitioners of complementary (or natural) medical methods. We are seeing a return to the older, gentler, "whole person" approach to health and recovery.

Building Cancer Resistance, like the other books in the Healthy Body, Healthy Soul series, offers you natural remedies and simple but powerfully effective strategies, taking a whole-person approach to health. The strategies in this book *will* empower your immune system so you're better able to resist or recover from cancer.

This book is not offered as a substitute for support you may need from healthcare professionals such as general physicians and oncologists, or counseling from psychologists or qualified members of the clergy.

But this series is founded on one simple principle:

We are the ones most responsible for decisions about our care and well-being. And the more knowledgeable we ourselves are about what we can do to improve our health or combat an illness, the more likely we are to remain well or to recover from sickness.

Fortunately, there is a great deal we can do to care for ourselves and improve our total well-being.

This book is full of carefully researched natural remedies and simple strategies that are known to build cancer resistance. You'll find them very practical, inexpensive, and easy to use. What's more, as you read through the chapters, you will be able to create a whole-life plan that will benefit your body, mind, and spirit—boosting immunity throughout your whole being.

As you create the cancer-resistance plan that works for you, I wish you good health...in body and soul.

David Hazard
Founder of The New Nature Institute

1

You Can *Resist Cancer*

Chuck has been given only a 25 percent chance of beating the cancer detected during a physical that was to qualify him for new life insurance. The news nearly wiped him out at first. *One minute I was cruising along feeling pretty good,* he thought, *and now I'm facing the struggle of my life.*

When the shock wore off, Chuck felt a surge of determination. *The doctor said one guy out of four will beat the odds. I've gotta do everything I can to be* that *guy. But what can I do to make myself as strong as I can be and increase my chances of winning?*

Sharon has just received similar news. But it's about her sister—she has breast cancer. It might as well be *her* diagnosis, though. Her grandmother had breast cancer, and her mother and an aunt…and now her sister.

I'm not going to wait around till it's my turn, Sharon thinks. *I want to do whatever I can now to build my immunity so I can resist cancer before I get it. But there are so many claims about products and techniques that "beat cancer." How can I know what's hype…and what really works to build cancer resistance?*

Every day we hear stories about people who *do* "beat the odds" and resist cancer.

Many of these accounts are dramatic, starting with something like this: "The doctors said there was nothing more they could do for me…"

Often, the turning point is the discovery of a "key" that changed everything. *This* guy, who was given no chance, decided he was going to arm himself with a positive mind-set and enjoy life to the max—and he's *sure* that was the major factor in his victory. *That* woman put herself on a strict macrobiotic diet and stayed healthy, while her siblings were not so fortunate. *Another* woman swears an herbal tea cured her in weeks. *That* celebrity claims she visited a New Age shaman who freed her from "a bad aura picked up during a past life" and the disease is now disappearing. *That* guy on the Christian radio program insists he was healed when he learned "how to let go of hostility and forgive."

A few of these claims sound pretty "edgy." Definitely *out there*…and definitely not for us. But many of these testimonials leave us with real questions:

Do any of these things really work? Would one of them help me resist cancer? If so, which one?

The Natural Approach

There *is* great news. Many discoveries are being made about the simple things we can do to resist cancer.

Such discoveries include the use of diet and natural supplements; physical, mental, and spiritual practices; and even the important place of supportive relationships in boosting immunity and blocking diseases—even major diseases like cancer. These discoveries are being made in a field now known as complementary, or natural medicine—a field founded on simple concepts.

First, the human body was created with its own systems for fending off illness and disease. As humans, we have several parts that make up our total being—body, mind, and spirit. To support overall wellness, we need to find and do what's health promoting for all aspects of our being. This creates a whole-person sort of balance in which each aspect of who we are supports and encourages the health and well-being of every other aspect.

Sometimes descriptions of this natural, whole-person approach to wellness are a little off-putting to Western, contemporary people who are used to relying solely on traditional medical practices as a means to good health. We're trained to listen for pinpoint diagnoses that come with a definite and aggressive treatment plan. We want to know exactly which drug to take to knock the problem out of us. But the simple fact is that, sometimes we *do* become overwhelmed, usually by living out of balance in some way that brings undue stress on one or more aspects of our being. And this state of imbalance and stress creates conditions that contribute to poor health.

For instance, overworking in our career may tip the scales. Under the pressure of a constant grind, we overproduce stress hormones, severely taxing our body. Then we may ignore recreation and a healthy physical regimen that would reduce our stress. Or, ironically and in the name of "fitness," we cram a workout into an already overloaded schedule, pushing to finish "on time" so we can get on to the next item on the agenda...unaware that we're actually only stressing ourselves more. Along with that, we can also miss out on healthy mental practices that would relieve us of the tension that generates from between our ears when we're in conflict, radiating out via the nerve and limbic systems to our whole body. More often than not, we're also unaware of health-enhancing spiritual practices, which release those even deeper conflicts we carry when things are out of line at the core level of our being.

And so, overbalanced in one part of our life...completely out of balance in others...we create conditions in which we're overtaxed and undersupported. With the scales of our vitality tipped like this—with stress too high, and factors that would strengthen our natural defenses way down—it's easier for illness and disease to overwhelm and take hold.

In cases when we're extremely depleted, or when a potentially deadly disease is draining our vitality, aiming the best drugs and aggressive therapies in the Western medical arsenal at the problem often prove to be ineffective. No drug can override hormonal deficits created by a diet void of revitalizing nutrients, or resolve relationship tensions that stress and drain the life out of us. No chemicals or beams of radiation can replenish a spirit that has lost its will to live because it is hopeless, and without purpose and passion.

We Need the Best Traditional and *Natural Therapies*

What we need then—especially in building resistance to cancer—is a whole-person approach that supports overall well-being. We need the effective tonics and immune-boosting practices now being discovered—in some instances, *re*discovered after a long time of disuse—by practitioners of natural medicine.

This is *not* to dismiss the need for traditional Western medical practices—what is known as allopathic medicine. Cancer is an aggressive disease, resistant to treatment. We *can* benefit from the aggressive treatments of allopathic medicine. The problem with these treatments is that they can be physically depleting in themselves, as most people who have undergone chemotherapy, radiation therapy, or surgery can attest. This physical stress, coupled with an already-draining disease, can further rob us of the vitality we need to resist cancer.

For this reason, many practitioners of a more traditional healthcare—including physicians and surgeons, therapists, and nutritionists—are now recommending the use of natural strategies that create balance and support overall wellness in every aspect of our being.

In fact, the strategies known to the practitioners of natural medicine *do* complement traditional medical practices. And as you try them for yourself, you will find they are also a necessary and vital part of your efforts to resist cancer.

Creating a Resistance Plan That Works for You

Some of you reading this are living with cancer. You or someone you know has it. Others have experienced it up close—watched the struggle of a family member or a close friend—and you want to protect yourself from this disease.

This book will help you create a personalized plan for building that resistance. You'll find dozens of healthful strategies recommended by a broad range of professionals in healthcare and related fields—including doctors, psychologists, physical therapists, fitness trainers, nutritionists, herbalists, spiritual directors and counselors, and others.

Choosing the strategies that work for you will enhance your immune powers and improve your overall well-being. These are easy strategies and doable. Some are fun and will add depth to your life. All of them come from new discoveries about the immunity-enhancing power of:

- *healthy mental habits that release mind-stress and stimulate biochemical healing*

- *spiritual practices that lift life-crippling, interior pressures and revitalize our core being*

- *a cancer-resistant diet, along with right eating habits, that arms the body against free radicals and carcinogens*

- *"team" relationships—those that don't tax and drain, but support and build us*

- *natural supplements—including herbs and vitamins—that are proven to arm the immune system*

- *recreations and workouts that fortify us with energy and endurance*

- *creating a sense of total balance that makes us strong in body, mind, and spirit*

Each chapter of this book addresses one of these vital areas of immunity enhancement. And as you read, you'll be trying out your own personalized plan, using simple, natural techniques that are known to improve cancer resistance.

On one hand, the strategies in this book will help you with very practical tasks of physical, mental, and spiritual *self-care*—all very important in the contest for your health. Equally as important, you'll find that using these techniques will quickly improve the *quality* of your life, helping you rediscover the richness of living—even the sacred nature of life. As you begin to achieve both inner and outer balances, you'll find yourself more fully "alive in the moment."

Your Guidebook to Improving Overall Resistance

What you have in hand, then, is a guidebook to the natural way to build cancer resistance. Using the strategies found here can improve well-being in all areas of your life.

Because you *are* a whole person—with body, mind, and spirit interlinked—you will not find in these pages the offer of a "magic bullet." No single change…no adjustment in lifestyle…no natural supplement or tea…no miracle food or diet…no new way of thinking or praying…is known to be *the* secret to curing or resisting this disease. For that matter, no product, technique, or book can offer us guarantees when it comes to our health.

What this natural approach to building cancer resistance *will* do is:

✓ *offer you natural techniques and tonic remedies that are, by and large, free of the harsh side effects associated with pharmaceuticals*

✓ *empower your immune system to better fight disease*

✓ *improve your overall health and quality of life*

✓ *restore vitality more quickly, if other necessary cancer treatments have left you feeling depleted*

✓ *give you the wonderful experience of living in balance—a sense of overall well-being in body, mind, and spirit.*

Most critical to those who are resisting cancer, you will be helping your body's natural defenses operate at peak effectiveness.

And there is one more important benefit taking this approach will give you.

Take Back Your Power

The natural approach has at its core a belief in the personal empowerment you can experience through improving your self-care. This is because you're taking a more active part in choosing what works best, and what's healthiest in the fullest sense, for you and your life.

Too often, people facing a major health crisis feel as if the power to choose at all has been pulled from their hands. This happens when we allow experts to press decisions upon us…and when we ignore our own self-knowledge and intuitions. It is not that experts take power from us; we give it away to them by not participating in caring for ourselves, becoming knowledgeable and active on our own behalf.

Unfortunately, a sense of powerlessness most often leads to frustration, depression, and the overwhelming sense of being "victimized." Then comes depression and even darker interior states. Many people spiral downward for a long time, into a sort of bottomless fear and anxiety. This negative state of being *itself* further suppresses immune function, weakening the body and decreasing our ability to resist disease.

When the power to decide and take part in improving our condition is given away—when we abdicate and hand ourselves over to be the responsibility of "experts"—we often do great damage to our ability to be resistant.

We need to work on our own behalf. When we take back a good measure of the power to choose and to do for ourselves, we literally begin to take back power to improve our condition.

For that reason, this book is offered to help you take up the necessary part you can and *must* have in drawing up a total plan for cancer resistance. Here is how you should use what you find in each chapter:

First, use the strategies in this book to improve aspects of your life where attention to self-care has slipped.

Some of us have never taken very good care of ourselves. We've put others first, or just ignored our health because we've generally felt good.

Others of us have paid attention to maybe one aspect of our health, like dieting to stay trim…but we're weak in another area. Maybe we have few, or no supportive relationships, or we've failed to develop a healthy spiritual life, or we rarely take part in revitalizing physical recreation or workouts.

Then there are those of us who have abused ourselves—maybe *directly* through substance abuse…or else *indirectly* through a poor diet, or staying in a job that's crippling to our sense of purpose, or never resolving relationship problems that crush our spirit.

Most basic to health is the attitude that says, *I am worth caring for. And it's worth it to spend my own efforts in taking care of myself.*

Each chapter presents a whole range of strategies, requiring lesser or greater commitment. You'll begin to recognize areas of your life wherein self-care has slipped. By adopting some of the suggestions from each chapter, you'll be boosting your resistance to cancer *and* making a renewed commitment to self-care.

Second, use this book as a tool to bring your life into healthy balance.

Life *does* work better for us when we live in balance. That is, when we cultivate healthy physical, mental, and spiritual practices.

Our tendency is to gravitate toward aspects of life where we feel competent and comfortable and to avoid looking at areas where we know change is needed. We don't like the discomfort of change or the uneasiness of feeling like novices and learners.

This is to say…you may need to avoid the temptation to skip chapters that touch areas of living you'd rather not look at.

For example, you may toy with the idea of flipping past the chapter on diet. You may instinctively sense it might mean making changes in the kinds of food you eat and your eating habits—and making dietary changes isn't easy for you. Maybe you have the idea that eating a healthy diet means eating mostly green leafy stuff—"rabbit food"—and you're not about to turn yourself into a rodent for any reason.

Which is *exactly* why you need to look at *that* particular chapter. It will not push an exotic or extreme diet on you. Instead it will show you how, with the addition of some simple strategies, you can turn normal meals into good-tasting, immune-boosting meals. At the same time, those who are willing to experiment will find some intriguing information about foods they may wish to try.

So if you feel like avoiding a chapter—*don't*. More than likely it's full of life-supporting strategies you need to bring your life into greater balance and to build your personal cancer-resistance plan.

Those who successfully resist cancer, and those who enjoy the best quality of life even during long and challenging treatments, are the people who have found a well-rounded balance in life that works for them.

Third—if you have cancer now—use the strategies in this book in combination with the treatments of healthcare professionals.

In the interest of building your own support team, you *will* need the help of physicians and also the aid of others who are experienced in various caring and fitness professions.

The best plan for resisting cancer will be to use the aggressive approaches of allopathic medicine in combination with the gentler, boosting, restorative approaches of natural medicine.

Doctors will provide you with the necessary scientific expertise and practical case experience. And they can provide medical testing that tells what your needs are, which treatments are helping you, and which are not helping. Obviously, they can also prescribe pharmaceuticals, design treatments, and keep you abreast of the latest discoveries in cancer research. You should also check with your physician first before trying certain strategies offered here.

Most definitely, you must tell your doctor if you decide to try any of the recommended herbs or other natural supplements. Certain herbs and supplements will react negatively with particular drugs. And even generally helpful supplements can affect the metabolism and effectiveness of pharmaceuticals.

To be very clear: Sometimes there exists an antiestablishment feel in books about natural healing. That spirit doesn't exist here.

Yes, it's true that some physicians are skeptical about natural medicine; there's good reason for that. Doctors in practice now were mainly trained in the scientific traditions of Western medicine, which includes giving long periods of study, observation, and testing to a treatment before declaring it effective and suitable for human use. Natural medicine, in its recent incarnation, is still fairly new. Many of the claims about the effectiveness of natural supplements, or complementary treatments, come from anecdotes—in doctor's lingo, "hearsay." In many cases, tests are just now underway to determine the effectiveness or ineffectiveness of many natural treatments, and also whether there may be side effects that will appear later.

Nonetheless, more and more medical schools have been offering training in natural medicine and complementary techniques. And new doctors, and some who have practiced for years, *are* beginning to encourage the whole-person approach to wellness and the use of self-care strategies that complement traditional medicine.

Occasionally you'll encounter a physician who still believes natural medicines and self-care therapies are useless…or who will not allow you to make choices that do not come from his or her menu of traditional medical techniques. If you're currently being treated by an individual who has this attitude, it will be up to you, of course, to decide whether to remain under their care and direction or not.

It is always in your best interest to find the healthcare professionals who fully inform you about the treatment plans they propose—and who will support your choices and work with you as you make self-care strategies an important part of your cancer-resistance plan. These men and women will play a crucial role on your support team.

Back to Balance

Earlier in this chapter we discussed the need for balance. We saw how we can live out of balance and tip the scales of health against ourselves. More needs to be said about this before we turn to the strategies.

The fact that we *do* require balance to live well and to resist disease offers us two sides of the same truth.

On one side, we've seen that sometimes the way we live can open the door to illness. But we must quickly add that the specific mechanism that triggers cancer is still unknown. And along with that, nothing is served by telling ourselves that we've contracted cancer because of something we did or did not do...or listening to someone else who tells us our suffering is our own fault.

Beating yourself up emotionally, if that's your tendency, is a waste of time and also uses your energies unwisely.

On the other side, if we can tip the scales against our well-being...we can also tip them back in our favor. We can recognize parts of life where we've lived out of balance in unhealthy ways.

Using this book as a strategy guide will give you a great start in restoring balance.

2

The Power of a Healthy Mind

John Milton, one of history's literary masters, said: "The mind can make a heaven of hell, or a hell of heaven."

Milton was referring to the mind's power to pick at flaws within the best life has to offer—or, on the other hand, to find a single element of transcendent beauty, truth, or meaning even in the most terrible circumstances. He was speaking of the mind's ability to determine our interior "weather"—our mood and outlook—depending on what we choose to focus.

Milton knew what practitioners of natural health practices have rediscovered today: The mind does have some amazing abilities. On one hand, our mind can actually work *against us*, making us anxious or compacting frustration until we're supercharged with stress, like so much powder in a ticking bomb….or it can work *for* us.

Depending on how we direct the focus and actions of our mind, we can actually add to our illnesses. Or the mind can play a very important part in boosting our immune function and creating a total, cancer-resistance plan.

Mental Stress

Most of us know our immune system is busy fighting off attacks that come from outside us. Bacteria. Viruses. We may also know it's working constantly to deal with attacks from within—for instance, working to eliminate damaged cells, including those that are precursors to the cellular chain reaction known as cancer.

But many of us are unaware that there are other forces at work against our immune system, wearing down our defenses. One of those forces is mental stress—an invisible enemy of immune function.

Mental stress is invisible to us because, as adults living in a challenging world, we simply learn to accommodate stress and tension until we can no longer see what we're doing to ourselves.

There are several ways we can do this:

One way is by rationalizing it—telling ourselves, *Everyone's got problems. So what? That's life.*

Another is by ignoring stressful situations, thinking, *If I don't make a big deal out of this, if I don't look at it, maybe it'll just go away.*

A third way is by carrying the vague if unrealistic hope that someone else will come and resolve stressful matters for us. Of course we're rarely aware of the underlying reasoning that sponsors this kind of false hope, which goes something like this: *It seems like too much work to resolve these difficulties. And I don't think I'm capable of doing what it would take.*

Unfortunately, as a result of accommodating stress, we've given it way too much room in our inner being. Many of us are what can be called "stress batteries," because we store up stress's negative nervous tension.

Mental stress can make our lives a living hell, just as Milton observed. It wracks our head with thoughts that pull in different directions. It torments us with negative thinking until all we can see coming our way is "the worst." It spills over into our spirit, clouding everything until all the darkest moods have benighted us.

The Mind-Body Connection

And then, of course, there is the profound effect mental stress has on our physical being.

When we're stressed, our body releases *cortisol* and other stress hormones. These are the chemicals that prepare our body for a "fight or flight" response. In stress-mode, for instance, blood is diverted from our cardiovascular and pulmonary systems to the muscles. Blood pressure elevates and breathing gets shallow. Other biochemical reactions, which are responsible for such things as healthy cell growth and the repair of damaged cells, are suppressed. In layman's terms, the body is too busy preparing to defend from an outside attacker to work on internal defenses.

In this way, mental stress triggers real physiological changes that profoundly affect immune functions. If we're under stress for a long period of time, our immune system can reach a state in which it's severely suppressed, functioning at the lowest level.

IF YOU ARE DEPRESSED

∽

Serious illness, or even the fear of it, often go hand in hand with depression.

Depression itself has seriously negative effects on our health. We can do great harm to ourselves by denying, minimizing, or just ignoring depression.

Some of the strategies in this chapter will help you to cope with depression. Nonetheless, you should make your doctor aware of your condition and get his or her advice and help immediately.

To experience an onslaught of depression while you're trying to focus your energies on resisting a major illness is like waging war on two major battlefronts at the same time. It will only weaken and wear you down.

If you are depressed, pick up a phone right now and call your doctor...

Using the Mind's Great Abilities

On the other hand, the mind has amazing capabilities that we can use to empower the immune system and improve resistance to cancer.

This is not to suggest that you can exert some kind of mental force and strenuously, energetically push back against disease. Nor is it a claim that you can open your mind and "tap into divine power"—as does a sales brochure that came in a mass-mailing, offering cassettes from a New Age "counselor" who promises to teach us all "how to work miracles." It's unfortunate that people who are facing life crises—no doubt some with cancer, and desperate to try anything—will likely send $39.95 for these tapes. Unfortunate, not only because they will be wasting their money, but because they will also be hoping for magic, or something very much like it, when they already have at their disposal the mind's true capabilities to resist disease and promote healing.

Actually, the mind's great value to us in immune boosting comes from this fact: By using certain, simple mental practices we can *release* mental stress and the interior pressure it creates on the body, suppressing immune function. Learning these simple techniques begins the work of bringing our whole person back into balance by restoring mental well-being.

The Mind-Body Strategies

Most of us are unaware of the simple, easy-to-learn mental strategies that promote good health. Some of them can be made as much a part of your daily self-care regimen as bathing or brushing your teeth. Others you can use to quickly de-stress when immune-suppressing tensions come arrowing at you out of the blue.

Some of these techniques will seem useful to you right away, others less so. Try them all, because you're likely to need each one at some point.

Strategy #1: Open the Mental Pressure Valve

One of the easiest mental stress-relief strategies can be done virtually anywhere, at any time, and costs nothing. Once you learn this technique, you'll understand why sometimes the simplest things in life are among the best.

Learning how to "open the pressure valve" mentally is *not* the same as opening your mouth and blowing off emotional energy verbally. All we do then is pass on bad feelings and stress to someone else, scorching a relationship as we do.

How to do it:

1. Identify stressful thoughts.

Stress occurs when our thoughts revolve around something that's frustrating, paining, or saddening us. In fact, we quite literally go around and around the problem, turning it over in our head—usually because we see no good way to resolve the issue. As we turn the problem over again and again with no resolution, we also intensify the negative feelings we're having about it.

Stress can also come from a period of intense concentration on any given subject or task, not necessarily just negative ones. We bear down on a long, long list of things to be done and intensify our mental energy.

In short, *prolonged mental intensity creates physical stress.* While we're consciously fixated on a given subject, all our nerves and muscles are in tension too. Perhaps you've been riveted on an intense drama on television. It builds and builds and…cut to a commercial. You realize your shoulders have been tensed, and you've almost been holding your breath.

A picture of how mental focus works can help you understand how to use this strategy. Picture intense, stressed thinking like this:

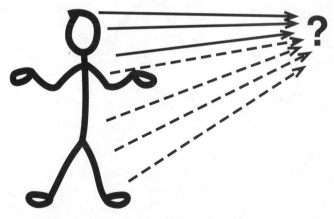

When we're experiencing mental stress, the strain on our physiology is very high. And we need to remain alert to thoughts and situations that trigger an overfocus on negative and intense thinking.

Are we overly occupied with someone's negative comments? Do we obsess about money, appearance, our job, or a relationship? Obviously, if we're dealing with a serious illness like cancer, our thoughts are likely to intensify on our illness and all the related concerns. And so our nervous energy keeps running like an motor left "on" much of the time. This state of being *will* run us down and deplete our immune functioning—unless, when we catch ourselves involved in stressful thinking, we do something to neutralize it.

2. Release your thoughts.

Fortunately, there is another kind of thinking we can turn to that will release mental stress. It's a kind of thinking that occurs when we're in a relaxed or serene state.

Quite possibly, you've relaxed under an open sky and let your eyes wander off into blue eternity. It may help to picture relaxed thinking like this:

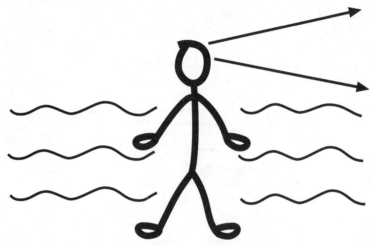

As we broaden our focus, mental energy becomes less focused and intense. As a result, our whole being automatically starts to relax. Muscles loosen. The heart slows. We breathe deeper. (Try it. Notice how quickly you yawn. You're expelling much more of the carbon dioxide that's been trapped in your lungs and taking in more oxygen.)

Focused beyond the boundaries of ourselves and our immediate problems, we're relieved of pressure. Tension drains. We've just released our mind and our body together, allowing them freedom to wander out beyond our present demands, limitations, and conflicts. With nothing on our minds, we can experience restfulness and a deep sense of well-being.

And now—the *really* important part.

3. Daily, practice letting yourself walk out of unhealthy mental stress...into healthful relaxation of the mind.

It really is a simple matter to train ourselves to switch from intense and negative thoughts to relaxed thoughts. Here are easy steps to use in retraining your mind:

- Make a contract with yourself right now. The contract says: "The next time I catch myself feeling stressed, I'll stop...and give myself a break. I owe it to my health and well-being to do this."

- Add to the personal contract a clause that says, "Every day, for at least five minutes, I'll practice these easy steps":

    ✓ Let your eyes come to rest on a distant point—for instance, a tree or the horizon. Focus on it for a moment...just long enough to transfer your attention from thoughts about the day's demands or problems you may be carrying. You can do this by noticing the texture, shape, or color of what you're looking at.

    ✓ Then allow your gaze to move up and off into space, into the open blue air or into a bank of clouds.

    ✓ Breathe in slowly through the nose and fill your chest. Breathe out slowly through the mouth. Allow your breathing to settle into a slow, deep pattern.

    ✓ Notice if there is muscle tension anywhere in your body. Relax the muscles.

    ✓ If any thoughts come, don't engage them...gently turn them aside. Allow your mind, like your vision, to rest "out there."

    ✓ If particularly troublesome thoughts keep returning, you may need to take a moment to jot them down. "Capture" them on paper where you can return to them later. Again...let your focus move between your breathing and the nonfixed open skies.

> **Note:** You can use this relaxation technique any-where—inside a windowless building, or while stopped in heavy traffic...even lying in bed at night—just by making a simple adjustment.

✓ Begin by shifting your attention to your breathing. Feel the way the air is cool coming in your nostrils. Enjoy the good feeling of filling your lungs and expanding your chest.

Benefits:

The more you practice this simple technique the more you will appreciate its many great health benefits. They are:

1. Relaxed thinking is a doorway to the instant physical, mental, and spiritual "downtime" we all need.

2. Wonderful chemical changes are triggered by relaxed thinking. The change that's touched off is known as "the relaxation response." When deep relaxation is triggered, our bodies release hormones responsible for cell and tissue repair, recharging our immune system.

3. Our bodies also release *endorphins*, those wonderful bio-chemicals that are responsible for giving us a sense of peace and well-being. Endorphins act like natural antidepres-sants—and keeping ourselves "up" is a very important part of making our way through any illness.

4. We open up a new mode of creative-possibility thinking. We seem more alert to life and more open to guidance, or wisdom that seems to come from outside our thinking.

Some would argue that as we experience deep, mental relax-ation we're just giving our brains a chance to connect facts and ideas it couldn't piece together while we were preoccupied or under stress. In short, we've given our brains a chance to arrange things in a sur-prising new order and come up with new solutions. Others would say we're clearing the way to listen at the deepest level of our beings which allows us to receive real spiritual insight. (We'll consider this more in the next chapter.)

In any case, many people who practice mental relaxation techniques insist it's during these times that they come to realize important steps they need to make to improve their health and well-being, or suddenly realize an important piece they've overlooked in their plan to resist illness.

Strategy #2: Get Into Flow Thinking

The previous strategy suggested a way to experience deep mental rest. A way to turn stress aside by dialing down the agitating negative energy it creates in us. This second strategy—getting into *flow thinking*—gives you a way to create and direct positive, healthful energies that exist inside you.

Flow is a state of mind and a state of being. It's what we feel when everything "resonates right" within us.

Flow thinking describes a state of mind that connects us to our dreams and creative impulses. As we act on these impulses, the energy of our *fascinations* join together with the energy of our *doing*... and real *creation* happens.

Artists and engineers...carpenters and neurosurgeons...at-home moms and corporate execs...anyone can experience times when they're in *flow*. Times when every fiber—body, mind, and spirit—feels energized and is moving in a healthy direction. *Flow thinking* leads to *flow acting*.

Far too many of us just go about our duties all day...then flop in front of TV...then go to bed wondering what all our toil has been for. Our whole being is unhealthily depressed. Finding out how to get yourself into *flow thinking*, and learning how to leave your own creative trail, is a combination that yields great health benefits.

We can enter into *flow* in different ways. See which of these ports of entry works for you.

How to do it:

1. Journaling.

To be truly healthful, journaling is best done with complete privacy in mind. What you write is for your eyes only. In this way, you can be gut-honest and allow your feelings and your thoughts to come out and unite.

Journaling de-stresses the mind. It gives order to our reasoning. It's a safe place to express tangled, difficult, suppressed emotions, a private stage where our most important dreams can come out and begin to grow. Too often, thoughts and feelings, dreams and intentions, are all a jumble. Physical, mental, and spiritual energies are like teams of horses, pulling us in different directions. We don't know what to think, feel, and believe about things…and so we don't know what to *do*.

One writer has said, "Writing *rights* things." Journaling can *right* things for you by getting thoughts, feelings, and values to line up. As our inner priorities right themselves, our deeds right themselves too—until we are living and acting more and more in accordance with our strongest values and passions.

2. Play.

In our culture *play* is greatly undervalued. We think the only play that's healthy is the kind that provides vigorous exercise and builds muscle tone. We ignore other important aspects of play and its ability to get us into *flow* and stimulate immune function.

For you, play may be…playing music…or playing an imagining game with children. The important thing is that it be play for play's sake—and that we *not* be in competition. (This in itself is a major switch some of us need to make.) What we're after is to climb out of the buttoned-down, "stress suit" adult demands put on us…and get into kidlike relaxation-mode.

When we play…forgetful of time and burdens…our bodies begin to direct energy to rebuilding and strengthening the immune functions.

3. Creating.

Creating gets some of us into *flow* faster than anything else. You enjoy running a hand-plane along the wooden trim of a table you're making. Or drawing house plans. Or laying out a garden. Designing a dress. Reorganizing a drawer, a room, a company. Arranging flowers…or planning a community festival. Every creative act we enter into lets our vital energies flow because we are tapping in to personal passions, reaping a deep satisfaction that gives our whole being a boost.

It's this rhythm and balance—conceiving of something, then using our physical energy to bring the idea to fruition—that stimulates our vitality and boosts immune response.

4. Caring.

Caring is really another form of creating, and it also brings many of us into the experience of *flow*.

One older woman with cancer who helps and counsels unwed mothers says, "When I'm holding a young woman's new baby in my arms, I have this incredible sense of peace and well-being. I feel like I'm connected with every other mother…and holding all the children in the world."

A young man with cancer reports: "I really care about little kids. I coach peewee baseball because, deep inside, I love to see these little guys light up when they connect with the ball for the first time…and learn to spit like the other guys. It gives me a feeling of satisfaction nothing else offers."

Benefits:

Getting into *flow thinking* has health-promoting benefits.

1. It reconnects us with our deep enjoyment of life and with the will to live—two great sources of positive vitality to have on our side when resisting an illness like cancer.

2. We experience being at one with something we love to do, and sense that we're following the natural course of our lives…exploring and discovering. When illness distracts us from our living, *flow thinking* leads us back to being fully alive in the present.

3. Because *flow thinking* ties us to expression, the things we're prompted to do and create leave a trail or a legacy we can be proud of.

Some who have experienced this realignment of passion and action—*flow*—and went on to recover from cancer often make remarkable statements, like this one:

I can't believe I'm saying this, but I'm actually a little thankful for the cancer now. It woke me up to the fact that I was living in a way that had nothing to do with my passions and values. Of course I'm grateful I recovered. But not just because I'm still existing. I existed before...but that's about all you could call it. Now, I'm alive. My life is moving on in the way it should be going now. I'm really on course.

Strategy #3: Thinking Through Barriers

Yet another source of mental stress comes from the sense that a circumstance or problem has trapped us.

A serious illness comes and we think, *I hate this...but I'm stuck with it.* Money crises arise, and we think, *Now I'm saddled with debt. Life is going to be all drudge work and bill-paying from now on...*

When we feel stuck, trapped, and our way seems blocked, we feel frustrated, ripped off, angry, and sad...and then comes depression and hopelessness. As our mental atmosphere clouds with depression, our immune response is suppressed as well.

To turn the situation around, we can learn how to "think through barriers."

How to do it:

1. Get the picture right.

We've come to a passage in life we've never had to go through before. Or maybe we've had this problem before, but failed to deal with it. In either case, the way on from here seems blocked by insurmountable obstacles. But we don't *know* that for sure. Our human tendency is to think there's no way *around* our problem, and no good way *through* it. Voices inside tell us, "Give up. You're done." Instead of listening to voices that say you're stuck, trapped, and blocked, take charge of the situation, like this:

Imagine yourself standing before a rugged mountain range... vast...blocking your way.

Sure, it *looks* as if there is no passage…but the truth is, there is no mountain range on earth humankind has failed to find a way through. So tell the voices of frustration inside your head, *There is always a way through every problem…including this one…and I'm going to do whatever it takes to find my way through.*

Now you've got the right mental attitude—the one that allows you to move on.

2. "Move closer" to the problem.

Examine it closely…all the options. Keep the imaginary mountains in your mind's eye. You are an explorer. Every explorer knows that hidden pathways and narrow passages—the way through—always reveal themselves…if you take time and look long enough.

When faced with a problem or crisis, most of us back off and check out mentally way too soon. Maybe we give in to fear or insecurity. We tell ourselves things like, *I'm not smart enough to figure this out. This is too complicated—way beyond me. Too much work!*

Explorers *keep* exploring their options. And a way through—however rugged, however much our mettle is tested—does open up.

Explorers also rely on seasoned guides. They don't go it alone; they ask around until they find someone who knows the particular mountain range they need to cross. (In doing so, they sometimes pick up wise companions who stick with them for the journey.)

3. Keep going…one step at a time…with the end in mind.

Okay, so this will sound like a bumper sticker slogan but: *The going may get tough, and you may have to get tougher to keep going.*

Whether resolving a problem or sorting through treatment plans for an illness…midway through a lot of mental effort most of us feel like giving up. Rather than quitting partway through…

Keep your mind's eye on the peaceful, beautiful plains…the wide open way…on the other side of the mountain.

What would the resolution to your problem *look* like? A healthy body?

What would it *feel* like? The resolution of anxiety and a return to peace of mind?

When the way is long and the challenges many, remind yourself that this work you're doing is just a means to a good goal. The reward lies beyond the mountainous difficulty…the one you're conquering, one step at a time, right now.

Benefits:

By learning how to "think through barriers" you're gaining in many ways. Here are some of the benefits:

1. You're relieving inner tensions that work against you by stressing your immune system.

2. You're sharpening yourself mentally, learning the powers of patient observation and reasoning.

3. You're toughening up emotionally, not giving in to frustration, sadness or anger…and the depressing sense of low self-esteem.

4. You're growing in spirit—growing in the "can do" attitude that gives us interior resilience.

Strategy #4: Making "Healthy" Decisions

Few things are more stressful than having to make crucial decisions that will greatly impact our life and our health.

Have you ever noticed that people who are decisive usually have a certain sense of calmness and poise…and a certain sense of deep-running vitality? These people hold several health-promoting attitudes:

→ *They accept that life is full of choices to be made…even difficult ones.*

→ *They understand that having a good decision-making process allows us to direct vital energy we need into life and good health.*

→ *They realize that we have to commit ourselves to trying something if we're ever going to find out if it works for us.*

→ *They believe we can adjust our course and keep trying new options if old ones don't work out.*

This combination of mental characteristics just listed—decisiveness *with* flexibility—is vitally important, not only to life in general but to help us as we determine the cancer-resistance plan that works best for us. The vast majority of us have "glitches" in our decision-making ability. We need to develop healthy decision making.

How to do it:

1. Recognize your present decision-making style...and the attitude that lies behind it.

Very often, a decision-resistant attitude blocks our way. We get hung up, fearful, frustrated. We check out and do nothing. Do any of these statements sound like something you'd think or say?

- *"I want someone else* [an expert, my spouse, my children] *to make the decision for me. Just tell me what to do."* You have a bail-out style of decision making. Your attitude is that others are smarter or stronger—more capable than you in *some* way—to make a choice.

Shouldering responsibility for ourselves makes us stronger and wiser in decision making.

Sure, we'll misstep sometimes. But we need to outgrow the fear that prevents us from deciding.

- *"Give me every option and every detail first. When I have as much information as I need to feel completely comfortable, I'll decide."* Your style is thorough...and that's good. But you may get hung up on gathering information. You may find yourself stalled in indecision because you're hoping a few more facts will "ensure" the absolutely right choice.

You can benefit by remembering you cannot make perfect choices. No imperfect choices makes you a fool or a loser.

- *"I know what's best for me. I'll make a plan... and let you know what you can do to support me."* The strong independence of these words may *sound* healthy and responsible. But we all need to recognize there are areas of expertise we lack and will never master.

You can benefit if you admit that, in some areas, others will have the authority of experience you'll never have. You'll benefit from bowing to their knowledge and allowing their experience to direct your decisions.

- *"I don't have to decide today. I'll decide when I decide. I'm not sure how I'll do that."* Your attitude is…procrastination. You put off the inevitable until the inevitable decides for you. More than likely, you get angry or resistant when someone who cares about you—someone who has a stake in your future—tries to push you to decide. But then, you're also angry and bitter when the inevitable hits you between the eyes.

Your decision-making process needs a lot of work. You need to decide *how* to decide.

(Keep reading.) You need to think through your values and priorities. You need to determine risks you're willing to take and costs you're willing to pay. In short, you need to come up with a blueprint for deciding what would work for you…and stop putting yourself and everyone around you in a bind.

- *"Guarantee me that this will work and I'll do it."* Sounds cautious and reasonable. But nothing in life is guaranteed. Certainly not our health. When we insist on guarantees we're asking someone else to play God. That never works.

Your decision-making process can benefit by giving up your need to have someone to blame and by allowing for the fact that everything in life has an element of risk.

2. List your values.

When we know our priorities, making choices becomes easier. When we determine what's most important to us, we also gain… determination. Raw willpower.

For example:

A young husband and father who is ill may determine that recovering health so he can be there for the sake of his family is his top priority.

An older woman may decide that it's most important to her to stay as available to her children and grandchildren as possible, to experience every day with them as much as possible. Being "present in the moment" is her top priority. So she may determine to use only treatments that have no side effects that would cause her to lose days or weeks resting and regaining strength.

3. Post your decision, so you and everyone else knows exactly what it is...and that it's based on what you value most.

Have you ever caught yourself "hemming and hawing"? Ever made a firm decision...then doubled-back on yourself...felt frustrated, a little foolish, and lacking in power? (Who hasn't?)

A decision is like a "base camp" on the journey of life. When you make a decision based on a priority, you stop moving your "base" around. To help solidify your choice, you may want to write out your reasoning for your own benefit...and also communicate it clearly to others as well.

Once you choose a top priority, you have a solid base from which to work in determining your next step. The woman and man above, determined to recover, will have great energy at their disposal to make their next moves, which might include:

→ researching their illness thoroughly, and all known treatments

→ locating practitioners of both traditional and natural medicines who can help

→ getting this team to strategize together, so a full range of complementary treatments can be coordinated

→ drafting a support team...people who they call on to keep their spirits up, maybe even push them supportively if the going gets tough and their determination falters

4. *Adopt an attitude of flexibility.*

As you read the attitude assessments in step one above, you probably noticed there are shifts you need to make. *Attitude adjustments.*

The ability to recognize our self-defeating attitudes is one of our mind's greatest powers. The attitude we have at one fork in the path is not necessarily the attitude we need at another. How foolish then to stubbornly cling to one attitude no matter what the situation. Sometimes we need to be stubbornly determined, but sometimes we need to give in to someone else's experience and choices for us.

It's a mark of great maturity when we use our mind's ability to *change our attitude.*

And when it comes to decision making, the supreme attitude we need, the one that governs all the others we might choose, is an attitude of *flexibility.*

Becoming flexible in our decision making will give us:

- a willingness to try new solutions, even ones we rejected before

- patience, to allow for missteps, and quick course changes when necessary

- the ability to sidestep mental "bogs"—like perfectionism, blame, complaining, and self-pity—and keep moving ahead

- the wisdom to ask for help and guidance when necessary

- the humility to submit to others' expertise

5. *When you choose a course, go with it...and don't look back.*

There are two parts to this step, but they act as one:

- *"Go with it."* A demand for 100 percent guarantees will hold you back. Remember, there are few guarantees...only more course adjustments. Moving into a choice is like staying for a little while in a city where you're thinking about moving...

you can't tell if it's going to work for you until you're trucking around the new streets.

- *"Don't look back."* Well, okay…you can look back *a little*. Hindsight is a great gift, but only if we use it to readjust where we're going. But *not* when we use it to torment ourselves with where we *could* have or *should* have tried something else. Remember, we don't have the godlike ability to know if different choices or other advice would *really* have helped us more or not. And blaming ourselves or others wastes time and energy we need for making new decisions or for revising our plan.

6. As your situation changes, keep revising.

Remember *base camp?* Following our example, a bedrock determination to do whatever it takes to recover keeps you steady. But you'll make choices along the way that don't work and aren't right for you. Remember the other half of decision making— *flexibility?* When one choice doesn't work out, revise your decision and try another.

Benefits:

A healthy decision-making ability keeps us involved in the choices, great and small, that determine our own well-being. Here are other benefits:

1. We learn how to take the lead on our own behalf, when knowledge, experience, and intuition tell us the way to go.

2. We learn how to take a step back and let healthcare professionals and personal supporters take the lead sometimes when we're in need of support or guidance for the next step.

3. We loose ourselves from the stress of procrastination, frustration, worry, and anxiety…and free up vital energies we need to become stronger and more resistant to illness.

Conclusion

Developing healthy mental practices is a vital part of a personal cancer-resistance plan. Unfortunately, these simple strategies are too often overlooked. Now you can make them your own.

Often overlooked, too, is the fact that mental health is fed by healthy spiritual practices...the way a spring is fed by underground wells of water. We'll turn now to strategies for creating spiritual health, which is another aspect of building natural cancer resistance.

3

A Resilient Spirit

*I*t's easy to recognize how a change in our physical body can affect our mind, even our spirit. Suffer an injury or illness that lays us low for a while and we find ourselves fighting restlessness and boredom. Suffer a catastrophic illness, and we're plunged into upheavals of frustration, anger, fear, and depression. We can feel abandoned, isolated. We ask questions about "the meaning of it all": Why *were* we put here? To go through *this?* And if so, *why?*

Body, mind, and spirit *do* interact, for worse...or for better.

Yes, for better. Though physical and emotional changes can affect our spirit, the reverse is also true. Changes in the spirit *do* have effects on our mind and body. And the right changes in spirit can have a most positive impact on our overall health and well-being.

For some of us, this is a new idea. But many people who have been diagnosed with serious illnesses have learned that the spirit plays a very important role in recovering health and/or vastly improving their quality of life. They've learned that when the spirit is made strong and resilient, it aids in resistance to even life-threatening conditions.

The question is, how do we develop a healthy spirit, one that gives us resilience from the inside out?

For those who may have come from the *Slap on a Cheery Grin* school of life, or the *Take It Like a Big Boy/Girl* school: We do not develop a genuinely healthy spirit by faking cheeriness or by stoically acting as if nothing's wrong. Wearing a mask is not the same as facing and dealing with real spiritual needs.

In this chapter we'll explore spiritual practices that will help build resilience from within—practices that are known to have spiritual, mental...and yes, even physical benefits.

The health benefits I'm speaking of are, in their own way, somewhat miraculous. Because developing a simple, daily regimen of these spiritual practices can:

1. trigger a deep-relaxation response, which in turn will

2. increase the production of immunity hormones, T-cells, and microphages

3. boost the production of neurotransmitter chemicals in the brain—those "feel good" endorphins that bring us mental clarity

4. promote deep respiration—good breathing—which circulates better-oxygenated blood

And on another important tack, these practices will also:

5. create more realistic and healthful relationships—with yourself, with other people, and with God

6. give you clarity and balance as your highest values become clear, and you begin to act on them

As I've already stated, citing the physical and mental benefits of good spiritual practices doesn't discount their value to your soul or to building a stronger faith. As a matter of fact, they will improve the quality and depth of such faith as you have. But along with that, they're highly beneficial to body and mind. And so in a moment we'll take a look at spiritual practices that make us resilient in spirit and benefit our total well-being.

But first, for those who aren't familiar with them, a word about these particular spiritual practices and where they come from.

Spiritual Disciplines

The practices we'll be looking at often go by another name—*spiritual disciplines.*

For many of us, the term spiritual disciplines is new. In Christian spirituality, this is a centuries-old term that refers to certain practices well known to strengthen and build health in the innermost being. As herbs are tonics for the body and mind, you could say spiritual disciplines are tonics for the spirit.

For purposes of this book, when I refer to spirit I mean: *the part of us that holds our deepest values, highest ideals, and strongest beliefs—the "code" by which we live.* This is the aspect of our being which, if it were activated and strong, would cause us to be our best selves.

Unfortunately, our spirit—like our body or our mind—can become weak and even sickly. It can be stressed with conflicts and confusion. Wracked with the pain of shocks and losses. And if we live in a way that ignores our values, ideals, or beliefs, it can sink into a state of atrophy from disuse. If we continue to live with stress, and conflict, cynicism, disillusionment, discouragement, or hopelessness at the core level of our being—that is, if we become weak and sick in spirit—we open ourselves to mental and even physical illness.

Many healthcare practitioners have witnessed the phenomenon of someone who is only moderately ill but whose weak spirit causes their health to become worse and worse. Conversely, many people with healthy, strong, vital spirits have conquered some of the worst illnesses—even surviving cancers that should have claimed their lives.

What we need in order to live well is a vigorous, resilient spirit, one that's full of vitality and that helps resist every kind of illness. But most of us have never had any training in disciplines that build such a spirit. With some practice of the strategies that follow, you can begin to develop a strong, healthy spirit.

Spiritual Disciplines for Health and Healing

These practices—some of them in use for millennia—have the proven ability to give resilience to the whole person. For that reason they are widely used by many people in the resistance of major illnesses including cancer. Some you'll recognize, but others may seem less familiar—or entirely new.

If you want to improve your resistance to sickness and disease, I highly recommend that you try each of them and make a place for them daily in your regimen of health-promoting strategies.

Strategy #1: Prayer

Maybe your idea of prayer is "asking for things." Or the recitation of someone else's inspiring words—like the Prayer of St. Francis, the psalms of David, the Lord's Prayer, or the Serenity Prayer. Or it's possible you have a somewhat more developed prayer life, one that includes offering gratitude or "praises to God."

But when we're faced with a serious illness like cancer, or even the threat of it, we're likely to find that new dynamics take over the way we pray. Suddenly, the old forms don't do it for us.

One dynamic is the sense that we need to *bargain*. We offer to do certain things in exchange for a clean bill of health. Another dynamic is the search for *power* or *leverage*. Maybe we ask: "Is there something I can say to God, or is there a certain *way* to pray, that will improve my chances of getting God to do what I'm asking?" Maybe we believe we've found a loftier form of prayer, and we simply offer a "prayer of surrender." That is, we passively trust God for "whatever happens."

When and if God doesn't answer these prayers the way we want, we're left at the mercy of one of two things—circumstances or our moods. Just when we hope we've struck a deal with God…just when we think we've "let go" of our life and handed it into God's care… something happens to upset our nicely set spiritual applecart. We feel we're back where we were, struggling with interior stresses. Over time, we may build up greater and greater frustration as we keep asking and asking…and the reply is long in coming…or what we get isn't what we asked for…or fears and worries return.

Here are two very old types of prayer. They offer profound and very practical health benefits for the whole person, which is why I highly recommend them.

The Prayer of Quiet

Many of us are unaware of the running monologue that goes on in the back of our mind all the time. We are constantly evaluating, commenting upon, judging, or making mental notes. And when we want to escape from our head, we turn on the TV, radio, or stereo and let *someone else's* thoughts flood our brain waves.

Constant head noise is wearying, even stressing. Some of us are, truthfully, intimidated by quiet because then we're confronted by fearful or unhappy thoughts and feelings. So we cram our days and our heads with sound. As a result, head noise stresses us constantly. We never give ourselves the opportunity to be still and rest at a deep level.

This constant head noise—including the sound of our own voice praying—has another negative effect on us. We feel lost and confused about important decisions we need to make. We unload and unload our questions…and remain confused. But we never quiet down long enough to see if a *new idea* might occur to us. True, we can experience rare moments when our mind is "out of gear"… and a flash of insight dawns. In that unguarded moment, a wiser voice from beyond ourselves seems to have spoken. But how often does that happen for you?

Practicing the Prayer of Quiet is a spiritual tonic, giving us a deep-spirit restedness. It counters the stress and intensity of life we carry, which wears us down physically, mentally, and spiritually…and also opens us to illness. This type of prayer also helps us listen long, until we gain a sense of confidence about important decisions we must make.

How to do it:

1. Find a quiet spot to be alone.

This can be a favorite chair by a window, or a rock on a wooded trail, or a park bench. "Quiet" and "alone" are the operative words.

2. Dedicate the time to God, and whatever sacred work might need to be done in you.

If God is the maker of our spirits, then God understands what our innermost being needs in a way that we do not. We are turning our will and intentions over to Someone wiser than we are.

3. Intend on being quiet.

Make it your sole intention just to fully experience the quiet. If you go expecting "lights" to come on or to "hear" a divine message, your mind will become active and intent on the wrong thing. *Ditto* if you're looking for a "mystical" feeling. Stillness, outside and inside, is the simple goal.

4. Bring a pad and pen.

When you try *not* to think about life's details, they'll clamor for your attention. Quickly write down the grocery item, the appointment, and the thing you must remember to tell someone, then gently turn your focus back to the quiet.

5. Make a transitional step.

When you're trying to find inner quiet is also when you'll notice even tiny noises the most. The hum of the refrigerator. Wind in the branches. Go ahead and focus on these sounds for a few moments…eventually you'll notice the stillness that's behind all sounds.

6. Enjoy the quiet inside you.

You may experience a buoyant sense of tranquility…and feel more alert and awake and alive than you've felt in a long time. Or you may experience a peaceful lull…such as you feel before falling asleep. (If you're overtired, like most adults, you may actually need to sleep.)

It's not uncommon, in this state, to experience a sense of the sacred, or the holy…and to sense that you are wordlessly in the company of God.

The Prayer of Quiet restores to us a clarity about our core values—about life, ourselves, those in our care, even things eternal. It rests the mind and gives it clarity for decision making.

And at the physical level, you will also experience deep relaxation. (More about this in a moment.)

Contemplation

Contemplation may sound otherworldly. The word calls to mind monks and mystics. But every day lovers practice Contemplation all the time. It's what we do when we fix the one we love in our mind's eye and dwell on all their best qualities. In a sense, we "take them into us" and let the fact that they are "ours" lift our spirit.

Most often, we let ourselves become overfocused on the gritty and the negative in life. On all these wonderful modern conveniences we own that keep breaking down. On relationships we depend on and which stress and disappoint us. From our inner being we sense a "flatness," even emptiness. A "who cares?" attitude takes over.

We need the restorative spiritual lift Contemplation gives.

How to do it:

Begin as you would with the Prayer of Quiet, in a secluded place. Then:

1. Focus on something that inspires in you a sense of... beauty, orderliness, gratitude, wonder, joy, holiness, love.

This might be an object from nature...or a special passage from the scriptures...or some aspect of God—say, God's creativity, gentle care, strength, purity, loyalty to us, or love. These qualities have another name—*graces.*

2. You might want to start by focusing on the grace of love.

We are loved at all times...whether our immediate circumstances are easy or difficult. And amid all the mixed circumstances of life, we have much to be grateful for...much that would show us we are loved...if we will but take the time to look for all its subtle evidences.

3. Focus on the evidences of love in your life.

It's one thing to meditate on some high, disembodied, spiritual concept like love. It's another thing to *notice* love…or the benevolent gifts of God…in the everyday stuff of our lives. We can notice benevolence…in the simple loyalty and constant care of a friend or spouse…in the companionship of a beloved pet…in the traits, gifts, and talents we were given to help us through life…even in the gift of life itself.

Note this: Contemplation will have the wonderful effect of helping you sense, not what you "should" be focusing on, but on what you *need*. (This is not about learning to "count your blessings.") Your own spirit will tell you what you're longing for in your everyday life.

For instance, you may find yourself contemplating not on love but on the graceful orderliness of nature. As this grand sense of order inspires you, you may realize your spirit is crying out for order…and that your life and relationships are too chaotic.

And so Contemplation—which we in the West have shunned as "too mystical"—actually leads us to a very practical next step (which is one of the main benefits of doing it).

4. Consider what adjustments you might make in your everyday life, based on the particular spiritual grace that has given you the lift you needed.

There is not much point, really, in having a lovely few moments thinking about a spiritual grace…like love or order or truthfulness…if it stops there. We have just experienced a profound connection with our deepest values…the qualities our spirit prizes and hungers for most. Now our task is to make a space in our everyday world for the spiritual reality we prize.

Ask yourself: How can I give and receive more love? What part of my life needs more order? In what relationships do I long for truthfulness?

Flow Praying

In the previous chapter, we discussed *flow* and *flow thinking*. Flow Praying is another form of prayer that offers important health benefits.

Flow Praying, to put it simply, is pouring out the raw contents of our spirit to God. It is simply opening up the stream of our conscious thoughts to the reality of God's presence with us.

Simple as this may sound, few of us do this naturally. Many of us "censor" our thoughts because we've been told, "There are some things you just don't say to God." Or we've been trained to use form prayers. It's as if God must be addressed nicely, politely, formally, or not at all. (If you happen to think this way, I recommend you read, for starters, some of the psalms of David, in the Old Testament, in which he rages against enemies, speaks of depression and despair, and charges God with failing to do what's right and just!)

Then realities of life come crashing in…and raw human need overwhelms us. A fear, a worry, an anguish. And our poor spirit is left twisting on a rope. At that moment some voice inside is reminding us not to say out loud what we're experiencing. This leads to something like a spiritual insanity—"insanity" being simply any type of gap in our reality: We're supposed to pretend we don't feel what we're feeling, and we're not supposed to react the way it would be normal to react. The deep-being kind of stress this creates suppresses the spirit, and the healthy functioning of the mind and body as well.

Flow Praying helps us connect our inward reality with our outward reality. It releases energy that's trapped and being used to ignore or deny stresses, and sets that energy free to work at healthful resolutions. Those of us who know the tonic benefits of this highly recommend it.

How to do it:

1. When you pray about something that's troubling you …stop and ask God to show you clearly what emotions you are experiencing.

One spiritual teacher has referred to this type of praying as "descending with the mind into the heart." For some of us the distance between head and heart is a lot bigger than the 18 inches of actual distance. We really are out of touch with what we feel…and so our thoughts and our passion exist in conflict. (If we doubt this, we should ask our spouse or friends if they think we're out of touch with certain emotions…but only if we're ready for a truthful answer!)

Take time to really notice what you really feel.

2. Pause, and ask to be shown clearly why your feelings are there. What's at issue? Are there two or more issues competing for the same space inside you?

Move even closer to the emotional content of your prayers. Often, more than one feeling is at work.

Because we're human, we are capable of experiencing several feelings at once—even opposite feelings. Grief and joy at a child's wedding. Relief and sorrow at the death of a parent who was suffering. Love and anger at a friend whose behavior is harming them and others.

Take time to sort out the different issues that are stressing your spirit.

3. Notice "censoring" voices.

Is some voice telling you, "It's terrible to be *this* angry with your parent…" or "with God"? Is a voice telling you, "You *shouldn't* be afraid?" "…angry"? "…sad"? Why not? "Because that's not mature"? "…Christian"?

4. Ask to be shown how to use the energy of your real emotions in productive ways.

Censoring our emotions is like locking powerful horses in confined little stalls. The idea is to let them out and get them harnessed in orderly fashion. If not, we turn our energies inward, where they become frustrated, developing into rage, depression, and deep grief.

We *need* to have the energy of our whole being available to us, to face life and solve its many problems and conflicts. Passionate energy—raw determination—is one of God's great gifts to us.

Asking God to show us *how* to direct our real energy opens us to the wisdom we know we need.

Benefits of these types of prayer:

1. Prayer is a tonic to the spirit. It immediately connects us with our Creator, the One who fashioned our being—body, soul, and spirit. The Prayer of Quiet brings rest to our spirit. Contemplation gives us a rejuvenating lift. Flow Praying benefits us by freeing our energies from the emotional eddies that prevent us from moving toward healthy solutions to our conflicts.

2. Mentally, we experience more clarity as a result of prayer. We begin to know what choices we must make to become more healthy and whole.

3. Physically, prayer brings a deep sense of rest…and oddly enough, more energy. Less energy is going into combating inner conflict. More of it is going into moving our lives in healthy new directions.

All three forms of prayer help us recognize the spiritual qualities we value…and which are lacking in our lives. We recognize that this lack contributes to the stressful sense that our life is out of balance, creating a spiritual climate inside us characterized by anxiety, grief, anger, or fear.

In terms of cancer resistance, the deep-relaxation response to prayer is what we need to trigger greater production of endorphins, which counter pain and give us tranquility. Deep relaxation also greatly increases production of the immune system's hormones, T-cells, and microphages, an obvious benefit in disease resistance.

Strategy #2: Spiritually Supportive Friendships

Sometimes we open ourselves to illness by living in tension, even opposition, with our deepest values. Maybe we've "drifted" into the position of being at odds with our own spirit, or maybe we've made a "bad choice" and feel there is no way to undo it.

Spiritually supportive friendships are important because they help us see the truth when we're living out of alignment with our own values, ideals, and beliefs. They help us answer the question: What *do* I hold as true and important? And then they support us in our efforts to realign what we say and do with what we believe.

In terms of our health, spiritual friendships help us move back toward a whole-being sort of resonance. Our innermost energies, thoughts, and actions line up again. Call it "spiritual chiropractics," or "living more at peace with ourselves and others," or "getting back in step with God." The end result is greater health and resilience in our core being.

Spiritually supportive friendships come in several varieties. Each one will have the effect of a "spiritual tonic," and will benefit your overall wellness. Those of us resisting cancer will discover some very important physical benefits.

The Confessional Relationship

The spiritual practice, or discipline, of confession may be completely foreign to some. For others it may bring back memories of intimidation and humiliation. With the right approach it has healthful benefits.

A confessional relationship is *not* necessarily one in which you just unload your faults and failures and then sit still for a stinging moral lecture. On the contrary, it can be one in which you unpack and sort out the various aspects of your life in the way you'd unload items that have gotten jumbled in a suitcase. The point is not to come away feeling judged, but to figure out your real personal convictions...and where you are living out of step with them.

A confessional relationship can help you to see the problems and dangers you get yourself into with your words and actions. It can help you see how you make little unhealthy choices that lead to big, unhealthy conclusions. In the end, a confessional relationship can help you understand how you needed to change your thinking and your actions to live in healthier ways.

How to do it:

1. Create a relationship that is "set apart"—one that's in a different category from all others.

Seek out an ongoing relationship with someone who is *not* going to be part of your everyday life. You aren't looking for a "chum." It's difficult to be completely open with a friend about your inmost troubles, doubts, angers, and terrors...not to mention humiliating secrets. Things said in this relationship are to be held in sacred confidence.

You might choose a member of the clergy or a professional counselor. Some rare individuals are also capable of handling confessional relationships, but be clear what you are coming to them for and what the terms of the relationship are.

2. Establish the terms that will make this a "safe" relationship.

Even if you're approaching a professional counselor, it's important to spell out what will make you feel relaxed and totally open. "Safe" to talk about anything. These terms might include such things as:

- total and complete confidentiality

- physical contact limits

- whether you prefer no religious terminology (if you're burned out on "God-talk")—or if you want spiritually based conversations only

3. Establish what it is you want to achieve through this relationship.

On the whole, you do *not* want to get involved in a confessional relationship with anyone who wants to make their personal agenda your agenda. Nor with someone who "needs to be needed." So *you* set the goals, which might include getting help with:

- identifying your spiritual code of values and beliefs

- changing the dynamics of stressful or unhealthy relationships

- gaining perspective on your life by receiving totally honest, or "more experienced," feedback

- realigning your words and actions—your *life*—with a value or belief you feel you've violated

To enlarge upon this last important point:

4. Work toward becoming completely honest about ways you know yourself to be in violation of your "spiritual code."

Every one of us has an interior "code"—a spiritual standard we believe is right. This may be as well defined as the Ten Commandments or not. It may also include "codes of conduct" we've picked up along the road of life—such as relationship ethics like honesty, fidelity, and self-giving.

One problem we encounter in relation to these inner laws is that we often come up with "good reasons" why we should *not* have to live up to our own code. These inconsistencies leave us in tension.

Another problem is that we are sometimes thrown into confusing circumstances that leave us conflicted. We don't know which value to use in determining our choices. Or we make one choice, thinking it's the best one...but later, in hindsight, feel regretful and wish we'd made a different choice. We live with the constant sense that we're "in violation."

The result is that our spirit continues to send waves of guilt-stress, shame-stress, regret-stress into our physical being. So in our core being, our spirit, we are crippled—never free to live and love life...maybe carrying the weighty, wary sense that a "hammer of justice" is going to come down on us. From there, spiritual stress affects our thinking. We become secretive, critical, down on other people and down on ourselves. (If we're going to live under the hammer, so are they!) And then these tensions translate into nervous energy, draining us of vitality needed by the immune system and eroding our physical well-being.

Very few people have no trouble at all being candid about their failures or "sins." Most of us have a lot of trouble with it—especially when the violation is enormous in our own eyes. A good confessional relationship will help us:

- recognize the part of our code we've violated

- take responsibility for our choice

- help us to be truthful about whether we made an honest mistake, or acted in a moment of weakness...or

- face facts, if we are intentionally, consistently acting in violation of our spiritual code, believing we can live without consequences

- encourage us, when possible, to right the wrongs we've done

Spiritual Friendships and Communities

Face a life crisis, like major illness, and suddenly we can feel profoundly isolated. Few people around us understand what we're facing, and we begin to feel cut off.

A sense of isolation or loneliness isn't just a problem of our socializing habits. Isolation is a main trigger of mental depression. A deeper sense of abandonment that depresses the spirit. This spreading depression engulfs the physical body, and we feel listless and tired. All the physical functions slow—including brain chemistry, metabolism, and immune response.

Spiritual friendships, or being part of a spiritual community, offer healthy, "tonic" benefits to the whole person—and one of the most important is relief from the sense of isolation that oppresses us, leading to illness or heightening the effects of an existing illness.

But experiencing the benefits of spiritual friendships or community does not happen automatically when you meet another person, or a whole group of people, who believes the same religious doctrines you do. Spiritual people can feel "lonely in a crowd" and not know why.

We must establish some relationship "terms" if we want to experience the health benefits of spiritual relationships.

How to do it:

1. Ask for support and help.

Asking for help may be one of the most spiritually healthy things we ever do. It puts an end to the isolation we impose on ourselves when we're being stubbornly independent and pretending we don't need help. We are not becoming dependent or giving others final control over us by asking for help. We're giving others a chance to know both our strengths and weaknesses…and we're helping ourselves by letting their strengths be added to ours.

2. Be specific in asking for what you need.

Do you need someone to drive you to doctors' appointments or treatments? Someone to just listen and let you talk? Someone to help you sort out options and choices—then stand back as you make final decisions? Someone to gently "crack the whip" and encourage you to keep going when you'd rather just "pack it in"?

Sometimes our relationships are disappointing to us and fail to help us where we need it for one reason only: *We expect other people to automatically know what we need or to guess—and they can't.* Voicing our needs is always our job.

When we're specific in asking for what we need, we set the terms of the relationship. And—miracle of miracles!—we're more likely to get the help we want.

3. Give the other person permission to speak to you about your "blind sides."

We can't know everything. We don't see all the possibilities. And we definitely don't see how we are occasionally our own worst enemies.

Sometimes when we're trying to make health-related decisions, we think we're making good decisions and we're not. Spiritual friendships can help us spot self-defeating behavior—but we need to give other people permission to address our issues.

This is as simple as saying, "If you see me doing something that seems like a big mistake, please tell me."

In this way we're inviting affirmation ("Good decision!"), as well as challenge ("Have you considered this option...?").

4. Especially—ask for a "lift" when you're down.

Sometimes we all need a ride on someone else's spiritual back. We need to be reminded, no matter how troublesome things look, that life *is* a good gift. Even more basic, we just need our friends to be present when words won't do it.

Sometimes we need to hear that we are doing the best job we can, given what we're struggling with. This can be even tougher than asking for help in the first place, but it really is okay to ask for emotional support: "Can you let me know when I'm doing a good job? Because I get discouraged, and sometimes I need to hear it."

Or we may need to ask for spiritual support. We may need to say: "When I get discouraged, remind me about the good things I've been given in life. Help me take my eyes off setbacks and focus on better things." Or: "When I'm really down, I don't think I can handle a pep talk. Just come and *be* with me, and that will let me know I'm cared for."

Benefits of these relationships:

1. When we release guilt and shame through confession we experience an overall "lightening up" in our being. We are releasing deep stresses we have carried. With this comes the release of endorphins, which block pain and give us an overall sense of tranquility or serenity.

2. Spiritual friendships and communities keep us from isolating ourselves and carrying emotional and spiritual weights that depress our whole being, wearing down our resistance to illness and disease. We are more connected to other people...and to life itself...improving an essential disease combatant—*the will to live and thrive.*

3. Spiritual friendships also provide us with a "sounding board" and practical counsel when we need to make complex or difficult decisions.

4. They may provide practical help with tasks we can't do for ourselves…making life easier at times when our health and well-being would be more taxed by the strains of living.

Strategy #3: Setting Healthy "Boundaries"

Many of us allow ourselves to reach a weakened and impaired state of being because we don't maintain healthy inner boundaries. We can literally run ourselves down and allow ourselves to become sick emotionally and physically trying to satisfy other people's needs and demands. If we have a major illness, like cancer, we need to establish firm boundaries in our lives to protect precious energy needed for disease resistance and healing.

"Boundaries" is a term widely used in psychological counseling these days. It simply means setting limits on how much we allow other people access to our time, possessions, thoughts…and to even deeper levels of our being, like our will. It means setting limits on how much of ourselves we give away.

If we have weak, or nonexistent limits, others are allowed to take from us freely…until perhaps we feel either overtaxed physically, mentally, emotionally, spiritually—or in all these ways. The result is that we become drained of vital energies, and we live with the unhappy sense that we are being violated by others' demands…and also frustrated and angry because we don't know how to stop them from draining us.

If we have well-defined inner boundaries, we do not let others have more access to us and our lives than we're able to give while still maintaining balance and well-being.

Spiritual Fortitude

Maintaining healthy inner boundaries is a new term for an old spiritual discipline. The practice of "spiritual fortitude," described by St. Augustine in the fourth century, builds "strong walls" that protect us from unwanted incursions which "unsettle the spirit and ruin its peace." In particular he warned about people who ruin the health of our inner being by the pressures and demands they place on us.

The spiritual discipline described here is similar to Contemplation—in that it requires mental focus, followed by action. This time, though, the focus is on looking honestly at our relationships and how they affect us. And then, of course, setting limits on the ones that weaken us…even suspending them if we need to.

If you have a hard time saying *no*…or knowing where "obligation" to another ends….and if it's draining the life and health out of you…I highly recommend this wonderful discipline.

How to do it:

Begin as you would with the Prayer of Quiet, in a secluded place. Then:

1. Picture your inner being as a city surrounded by a wall.

It's important to recognize that we have choices in life. Too often we tell ourselves we "have to" let others take from us, or we "have to" do for them. But in order to be healthy we need to set realistic limits in relationships—an ability that comes from being strong enough to say "yes" or "no." The wall represents the strength of your ability to do this in relationships.

As you consider the "wall" around your spirit, ask yourself: *What condition is my wall in? Am I able to say no when that's what I need to say?*

2. Consider the various people in your life who approach the wall around your spirit.

Get a clear picture of what they take away when they leave. Who are the people who make continual demands upon you? Friends? Family? Co-workers? What kind of drain do they put on you? Is it physical, emotional, spiritual—or a drain on resources like money, time, or possessions?

Some demands are clearly spoken: "Clean my clothes." "Fix my car." "Give me money." "Do this project for me."

Others are unspoken—by the friend or family member who just "assumes" you'll do for them, or by the boss who increases your workload without offering extra pay, or the person who dumps their bad feelings and leaves you distressed and down.

3. Consider the content of their requests and demands.

Are they reasonable or unreasonable? Are they asking you to do things for which they should be responsible? If they claim they "can't" do these things for themselves—or without your help—is that *really* true? Did you agree to help them at one time, but now it's past time for them to take responsibility again?

Ask yourself: *Do I take on too much responsibility for someone else's…finances, housing needs, personal care…or for their emotional, physical, or spiritual well-being? By carrying these responsibilities, am I really helping them in the long run?*

4. Consider the tone and manner of their approach.

Sometimes we even allow ourselves to be abused, manipulated, or just plain used by other people.

Is their tone angry and threatening? Or whiny? Are they violent? Do they take you and your help for granted? Are they just "takers," never offering any kind of fair payback?

It's time to face the facts if you aren't giving out of a genuine desire to give but out of compulsion—either to protect yourself or just to make them "happy." Time to face the fact that this is not a well-balanced relationship. And that you're draining yourself in some way, small or great, for someone else's benefit.

5. Be honest with yourself about why you take on others' responsibilities.

Often we blame other people for asking too much of us. And, yes, some people can overpower or wear down our "walls." More often, though, we have reasons why we open wide the walls of our spirit and give certain people unlimited access to us and our inner and outer resources.

Usually, there is some emotion at work that causes you to cover someone else's responsibilities. Recognizing it can be tricky, but if you don't do it, the emotional factor will continue to undermine your "walls" and they'll keep crumbling. (You may need the help of a spiritually supportive friend to see clearly why you give in.)

Ask yourself: *Why do I do it? What feeling would it bring up in me if I turned them down? What do I fear will happen if I don't do what they ask?*

6. Rebuild your "boundaries" by returning work and responsibilities to their rightful owners.

If you're going to redirect your vital energies to the work of disease resistance and healing, you need to return to other people the work they should be doing themselves. If you have cancer now, you cannot afford to expend energy sorting out others' problems.

You will need to take clear steps to transfer back responsibilities you've carried. You may need to write out a plan to help you stick to the new limits you're setting. You can even write yourself a short "script" if you need to. For instance:

- If someone's anger or threats have cowed you into doing what you don't want to do, get help from legal authorities to stop the abuse. It's time for them to be held accountable for their abusive words and actions.

- If someone is dumping work or negative emotions on you, it's time to say, "I no longer have the energy to do this job," or "I no longer have the energy to handle the stress I feel when you tell me these things."

- If someone is manipulating you ("Well, okay, if you won't help pay my bills I guess I'll just lose my car"), it's time to end the game. Time to say, "I don't have the resources to help you anymore."

Benefits:

1. We may turn unbalanced and draining relationships into healthy, spiritually supportive ones. Minimally, we stop the drain on our whole person.

2. By relieving ourselves of overwork and stress, we allow physical, mental, and spiritual vitality to be redirected into the

very real and necessary immune work of disease resistance and healing.

Strategy #4: Sacred Reading

In the third century, sacred reading emerged as a recognized tool to promote physical and emotional healing in a way that, as one writer put it, "sends all manner of evils fleeing." In the eleventh century, Hildegard of Bingen, an abbess and herbalist, also prescribed sacred reading for those who came to her seeking treatment for their ailments. And actually, the belief that sacred reading has healing virtues has been around since much earlier times.

But…*reading* in the service of health and healing? Consider:

Life's challenges are constantly wearing on us. Everyday demands grind us down. Trouble and evil in the world leave us with fear and anxiety. Circumstances catch us by surprise, and we lack the wisdom of experience to handle difficulties and complexities. We can feel bombarded and overwhelmed. *Add* to this the inner challenges we face with a major illness like cancer—roller-coaster emotions, for example, which alternate from hope to despair, from courage to fear, from determination to giving up and soon even the strongest person feels drained.

Sacred reading provides a steadying handrail for the inner being, keeping us balanced in spirit and offering health benefits.

Here are two types of reading you'll want to try as you create a regimen for disease resistance and recovery.

Scriptures

Although the Scriptures of the Bible are indispensable to the Christian, even the casual reader will find nourishment in the pages of this all-time best-seller. You will find many biblical writings that are refreshing for their honesty and authenticity about human experience—and for their ability to give voice to our deepest feelings, thoughts, questions, and conflicts. Mainly, for their ability to lift the spirit.

How to do it:

You will find many biblical writings that are refreshing for their honesty and authenticity about human experience—and for their ability to give voice to our deepest feelings, thoughts, questions, and conflicts. Mainly, for their ability to lift the spirit.

For a reading experience that's spirit lifting and healing, begin or end your day with selections like the following:

Psalm 6	Psalm 23	Psalm 31	Psalm 62	Psalm 97
Psalm 13	Psalm 27	Psalm 33	Psalm 66	Psalms 145-150
Psalm 16	Psalm 28	Psalm 34	Psalm 84	
Psalm 18	Psalm 29	Psalm 40	Psalm 86	
Psalm 20	Psalm 30	Psalm 47	Psalm 91	

Inspirational Writings

Many people of faith have faced illness, anxiety, and life's distresses and written to share with us the spiritually restorative wisdom they've gained.

Here are a few great writings that also have a tonic effect:

- *On Living Simply*, St. John Chrysostom (compiled by Robert Van de Weyer)

- *Abandonment to Divine Providence*, Jean-Pierre de Causade

- *The Love of God*, Oswald Chambers

- *Let Go*, Fenelon

- *Meditations on the Heart of God*, Fenelon

- *Revelations of Divine Love*, Julian of Norwich

- *The Problem of Pain*, C.S. Lewis

- *Miracles*, C.S. Lewis

Benefits:

1. The wisdom and faith of these insightful writings raise our viewpoint above our current circumstances by "opening our

eyes" to see life from a "higher" perspective—one that's based in spiritual, not physical, realities. This has a spirit-steadying effect that counters roller-coaster thoughts and emotions.

2. We experience a release from the stress of anxiety and a deep-being peace that stimulates physical immune response.

Some Warnings About Spiritual Fraud

A life-threatening illness can make us spiritually vulnerable. We tend to be much more open to anything or anyone that claims to have the miraculous ability to restore our health.

Spiritual convictions are highly personal and individual, this I know. I am not trying to discourage you from developing a more active faith. (Personally, I have witnessed both instant and slow recoveries from serious illness that cannot be explained by medical science and that only make sense in the context of faith.)

Nonetheless, experience bids me to warn you: Do not put your hopes in anything or anyone who promises you "perfect health," or "protection from disease," or "a miraculous healing"...*if* you will do one of the following:

- *give money, or turn over legal ownership of a house, car, or business*

- *pray a certain prayer a certain number of times*

- *attend a certain number, or kind, of religious services*

- *renounce family relationships*

- *quit trusting in the advice of medical professionals*

- *turn over your will or decision-making responsibilities to a religious leader*

Even people who would normally know better can fall for such promises when their health and life, or that of a loved one, is at stake.

Healings that cannot be explained by science come from the hand of a Being who is benevolent and knows all about us...and who surely does not need bribes or "proofs" of our faith.

4

A Cancer-Resisting Diet

Many of us have tried new fad diets that get a lot of media attention and hype—only to find the claims are overexaggerated. It's easy to become skeptical.

Is there such a thing then as a diet that can help you resist cancer?

The good news is *yes.* There are foods that have great potential to help prevent or combat this disease. The bad news is, if you're the average person living in the Western Hemisphere, you're probably not eating a cancer-resisting diet right now.

With the benefit of a little knowledge, though...plus a plan for making some simple changes...you can add the natural "medicines" in certain common foods to your overall plan for cancer resistance.

If you have cancer in your family history, you can help prevent cancer by making strategic changes in your diet. What you learn in this chapter will help you develop a diet that protects you from the effects of environmental toxins, and also from the biochemical toxins and breakdowns within your body, which can trigger cancer. And if you have cancer now, you can benefit greatly from the tumor-fighting, immune-boosting natural "medicines" in certain foods.

Many of the foods you'll read about in a moment will help prevent or repair damage caused by anticancer drugs and therapies, neutralize the toxins given off by tumors, *and* boost your immune system, helping it to fight not only the cancer but secondary infections: cold, and other viruses that can take advantage of a weakened physical state.

Before we look at the components of a cancer-resisting diet, it's important to consider our attitude toward food and eating in general—because attitude greatly affects what and how we eat. It also affects what changes we're willing to make for the sake of our own well-being.

Food as Medicine?

St. Augustine said, "I approach food as I approach medicine." This may not sound very appealing. In fact, it may sound pretty "monkish." It doesn't seem to leave any room for enjoying a juicy T-bone or a delicately flavored butter sauce. Forget a good wallow through a dish of "Calories Galore," that favorite dessert of yours.

Whatever else St. Augustine might have meant, his statement makes one thing clear—our attitude toward food *does* determine what and how we eat. And when it comes to food, attitudes are very strongly tied to emotions. Our heads may be strongly fortified with facts about healthy diet, but deep down inside we will resist making those changes if we're caught in the grip of even stronger, emotionally charged associations—*food-mood relationships.*

You would think that the prospect of improving our health, and possibly avoiding or helping to cure a devastating illness like cancer, would be big motivations for changing our eating habits. But no. When it comes right down to it, we human beings generally live by a life formula, which, put into words, goes something like this: I want to get the most benefits for the least effort and discomfort...Make that *no* discomfort.

For many of us, food has deeply rooted emotional connections. Because of that, any suggestion that we make changes to our diet can make us uncomfortable. And to most of us, uncomfortable = *bad.* One man at a recent seminar put it this way, with some intensity of feeling: "I'd rather die than give up my red meats." (Oddly, no one had suggested he give them up; he'd just been encouraged to consider healthier protein options.)

Here are some of the more common food-mood relationships you may need to work through as you try to change your dietary habits.

Food is a reward to me. This attitude may control your overall eating. That is, you may feel that eating in general is a way to reward yourself—for hard work, for being a good parent, you name it. It can also be attached to a certain food—a steak, ice cream, chocolate.

If food is your reward—if it says to you, "You're good and you deserve it!"—then you're likely to perceive cutting back, or cutting out, or changing, as a punishment.

Food is a comfort to me. For many of us, food is our most constant source of nurture and comfort. Even if we don't attach it to our performance—that is, to a good or bad judgment about ourselves—we associate it with being cared for.

Certain foods "tell" us we're cared for (for instance, cake) and others will not (okra). As it happens, comfort foods are usually those that contain sugar or quickly turn to simple sugar in the mouth. They trigger insulin production and a whole-body shift—from *work-and-use-energy-to-build* mode…to *relax-and-store-fat* mode. In short, they offer biochemical comfort. (Considering that most of us, unfortunately, view our work as "taking something from us," it's no wonder we come home from work and spend evenings reaching for "comfort foods"…and storing fat.)

If certain foods "say" comfort to you, then cutting back on them will make you sense a loss of being "cared for."

Food reduces my anxiety. Many of us feel anxious when we're bored. ("What am I supposed to *do?*") Or we feel anxious when things are uncertain. ("Will she get home safely?" "How can I pay these bills?" "Will he go out with me again?" "The boss seemed unhappy with me today…") Food, on the other hand, is stable. We can always count on a cookie to taste like a cookie. Some foods can also trigger the production of endorphins and other "feel good" brain chemicals that give a sense of tranquility and release from anxiety.

If the act of eating releases you from anxiety, or if certain foods trigger a biochemical "peace," dietary changes can leave you uncomfortably restless.

Food means nothing to me. I don't think about what I eat. I just eat what's put in front of me. This attitude is probably not entirely truthful. And if it is truthful, it's far too passive and neglectful. What it implies is that you and your body are just not important. If, on the other hand, you and your body are *not* very important in your own eyes, you'll do well to develop some determination and a fighting spirit. (Make sure you read the chapter on spiritual strategies.)

Perhaps the way you eat—carelessly—*is* characteristic of your approach to life. But you, your body, your health...your *life*...are gifts. You'll discover this if you stop treating yourself with indifference and neglect. Making changes for the better in your diet is a great way to begin honoring the gift of your life *and* the Giver of the gift.

As you can see, food-mood relationships have roots deep in our minds, and deeper still, in our spirits. But we can work ourselves free from self-defeating attitudes if we need to make important health-related changes in our diet. We can do so by:

1. Identifying food-mood relationships.

If you are serious about using a cancer-resisting diet, you may benefit by keeping a food journal for one or two months. Take note of the moods that trigger you to eat when you're not hungry. (What were you feeling? Bored? Anxious?) What did you eat? Also, take note of any mood swings you experience after meals and snacks. (Caffeine used to perk you up—but could it now be a source of your edginess and sharp tone? Chocolate comforts you sometimes—but could its high-fat and sugar content be dumping you into the blues at other times?)

2. Make a list of eating habits and foods that put you out-of-balance in connection with reality.

Do you stuff yourself when you're bored or anxious? Reward yourself with a huge steak or the most "sinful" sundae on the dessert menu? Comfort yourself with pasta and cheese...or cake?

What exactly *are* your mood foods? How sane is it to punish and overtax your body, and harm your health, in the effort to reward yourself emotionally?

3. Replace your old view of mood foods with a new view—until it becomes the new reality.

At one time or another, we've all arrived at certain views based on what we thought at the time were logical conclusions...only later to discover that those conclusions were wrong. So to replace an old view—say, about food—we'll need to do some work to update our thought processes. This means writing new scripts for the way we talk to ourselves about our mood-food foods.

For instance, in the past you may have said to yourself, "I finally finished the worst, most challenging project of my life. I'm going to go out and gorge myself to celebrate the victory. After that, I'm going to drink until I get a good 'buzz' going, because I need to relax and lighten up."

Then you learned that overeating, though rewarding your taste-buds, actually punishes your body. And that overconsuming alcohol is toxifying. How then is this a celebration? Because it's an illogical conclusion—one not based in reality—it's actually pretty insane, or at least foolish.

Today, you decide to base your new thinking in reality.

So you *stop* telling yourself you're being "punished" or "deprived" when you change your eating and drinking habits, and when you reduce or eliminate a certain food that needs to go. And you *begin* to tell yourself, "Now that I've finished this tough project, I'm going to celebrate by [doing something fun and stress-releasing]."

By practicing these simple steps, in time we gain a new mastery over our eating. Lo and behold, we find that we can actually take a healthful approach to eating. Maybe even, like St. Augustine, we can "approach food like medicine" when we need to.

This brings us back to the role of diet in resisting cancer.

A Diet for Resisting Cancer

What kind of diet helps us resist cancer? The answer is a diet rich in foods that:

➔ deliver a minimum of toxins from the environment

➔ deliver maximum phytochemicals (plant chemicals), which protect us from toxins—those naturally produced by our bodies, those given off by tumors, and those taken in during chemo- and other therapies

➔ do not stress our bodies by draining hormones and energy for digestion

→ help produce healthy red blood cells to carry oxygen throughout the body

→ promote the healthy reproduction of RNA and DNA, and healthy cell growth

→ help produce T-cells and microphages to boost immunity

Finally, a cancer-resisting diet—like any other diet—needs to be good tasting. If a diet is bland, who's going to stick with it? It also needs to be rich in variety. We need this to keep from getting bored and slipping back into old eating patterns that work against our well-being.

The following food lists will help you add more cancer-resisting foods to your diet. They are listed by food groups, so you can create balanced menus to suit your personal taste. Pay attention also to the percentages of protein, carbohydrates, and fat needed to balance your diet.

Protein

Certain types of protein are known to promote overall health. Others are known to stress the digestive system, tax our hormonal output, and circulate more acid and toxins throughout the body.

Before we look at which proteins are beneficial in a cancer-resisting diet, a word of healthy advice: In general we need *less animal fat* in our diets. Animal fat—especially red meats—will tend to contain higher amounts of omega-6 fatty acids. This acid is what we know as "bad cholesterol," and is known to promote tumor growth. Nutritionists recommend a balance of omega-3 and omega-6 fatty acids—collectively known as essential fatty acids (EFAs).

Many cancer experts highly recommend a vegan diet, eliminating animal ingredients altogether. Here in the Western Hemisphere, where we're used to eating slabs of meat as a main course, we tend to be unaware of the fact that we can get great protein from plant sources. (We'll discuss the other great benefits of plant-based nutrition as we go along.)

But if you love meat, don't despair. Here are healthy, good-tasting, and best choices to make for cancer-resistant eating:

Chicken. Though claiming to be the healthier choice, some chicken is actually loaded with unhealthy fat...while some is not. Read the labels. What are you looking for?

People who are conscientious about their health have switched to eating free-range chicken raised on grain containing DHA, which makes the meat high in both omega-3s and omega-6s, giving it a healthier balance. If chicken are fed with DHA, you'll find that information on the label.

Fish. In cultures where fish is the main meat source, studies have shown that people are healthier across the board. This includes a far lower incidence of cancer than in cultures that consume more red meat.

Fish are high in omega-3 fatty acids, and they contains other nutrients important in cancer resistance, including vitamins B_6, B_{12}, and folic acid.

What follows is a list of recommended fish and other seafoods, with those containing the most EFAs on top:

- anchovies, herring, mackerel, salmon

- albacore tuna, sablefish, sardines

- bluefin tuna, trout

- halibut, swordfish

- freshwater bass, oysters

- sea bass

- pollock, shrimp

- catfish, crabs

- clams, cod, flounder, scallops

Turkey. Again, you're after turkey that's been fed grain containing DHA.

An added benefit of turkey is that it's high in tryptophan, a natural amino acid needed for the brain's production of neurotransmitter chemicals. Studies show that when these chemicals are at low ebb, our moods swing toward anxiety and/or depression. When dealing with a major illness, the additional mood-boost can be important.

Eggs. The eggs from free-range chickens are your choice. Since they come from birds raised on the special feed mentioned above, these eggs contain a balance of omega-3 and omega-6 fatty acids.

Soy foods. As an excellent source of plant protein, a diet that includes a number of soy foods is a much healthier choice. Besides that, soy is a great source of genestein, a substance that blocks the flow of blood to tumors—in effect, causing them to starve.

Some of us remember the horrible-tasting soy products force-fed to us by an eccentric, hippie friend of our mom. (Personally, I used to refer to tofu as "toad food.") If your first experiences were disgusting to the palate, you'll be happy to discover that makers of soy food products have found ways to make them taste good. You can now find delicious products like soy milk, soy cheese, soy burgers, soy mayonnaise, soy sausage, soy bacon, soy yogurt…you get the idea.

Soy is also an ingredient in miso, a paste used in making flavorful soups and sauces.

Your protein goal. The goal of a generally healthy, balanced diet is to have about *30 percent* of your caloric intake from protein. And the goal, if you are creating a cancer-resisting diet, is to choose these proteins mainly from plant sources…or from animal sources high in omega-3 fatty acids…or at least from those that offer a healthy balance of omega-3s and omega-6s.

Need a Transitional Eating Plan?

If you're serious about cancer-resistant eating, but don't want to give up meat, try this:

- *Eat one meal a day that is totally vegan, including plant-source protein.*

- *In a month, add a second meal that is very low in animal fat…And a month later, switch to a plant-source protein, making it your second vegan meal of the day. (You'll probably have to add in a midmorning and midafternoon snack—say, fruit and activated yogurt—to keep the stomach rumbles down and your energy up.)*

- *Your third meal can be the meat meal. Choose from the recommended list above—and feel great about the way you're taking care of yourself.*

Think of meat as a side dish or a garnish…and you're on the road to healthy and cancer-resistant eating.

Carbohydrates

In general, a healthy diet is higher in complex carbohydrates, like fruits and vegetables, and lower in simple carbohydrates, like pastas and breads.

This rule—more fruits and vegetables, less pasta and bread—is important for overall healthy eating, because simple carbohydrates stimulate insulin production. Early in life, insulin helps the cells assimilate food nutrients for energy and cell reproduction. But in time, our cells become insulin resistant, meaning they turn away food energy. So the food energy is stored as fat.

If you're eating to build cancer resistance, getting your carbohydrates from plant sources is very important. That's because plants are rich in phytochemicals (and there are thousands of them), also in vitamins, minerals, and fiber—all cancer-fighting. And so are these powerhouse foods:

→ offer the antioxidant benefit of cleansing the blood of free radicals, those damaged cells that destroy other cells, sometimes triggering cancer

→ contribute to the duplication of RNA and DNA for healthy cell reproduction

→ stimulate the production of the immune system's T-cells and microphage cells

→ block the flow of blood to tumors

→ protect healthy cells and organs from toxins

Note: You need at least five servings of fruits and vegetables a day to get the cancer-resisting benefits of the phytochemicals in these foods. The old adage: "An apple a day…" will not do it.

The best choices, of course, are organically grown fruits and vegetables. They're not covered with wax, and they're free of toxic pesticides. Some carbohydrates are more highly recommended than others. Here are the ones most recommended for cancer-resistant eating:

Fruits. All fruits contain healthy nutrients and fiber. Fruits are also very high in antioxidant enzymes, vitamins, and minerals.

About Antioxidants

Because you'll be reading a lot about antioxidants in this chapter and the one on natural supplements, here is a brief description of the crucial role they play in balancing out a natural physical process that often goes awry and triggers cancer.

In the normal process of living and aging, cells wear out, and at the same time genes break down in the course of reproduction. This process of biological "oxidation" has been likened to the rusting, or corrosion, of metal. It is because of this process that damaged cells, or free radicals, are formed and cancer is likely to occur. Antioxidants are substances that bond with free radicals, preventing them from damaging still-healthy cells, until they are eliminated from the body. Many nutritional experts recommend eating fruits that are more ph-neutral or basic when you have cancer. Pay special attention to the advice about citrus fruits.

Here are the most recommended fruits and their cancer resisting benefits:

- **Apples.** Every type of apple you might enjoy is high in the superantioxidant quercitin. Apples are also high in fiber, to cleanse the colon. If "an apple a day" gets old and you want to switch to another ph-basic fruit you can buy year round, reach for pears.

- **Bananas.** An excellent way to replenish potassium and other important minerals leeched from the body during some cancer therapies. (Also a good source of thickness and fiber in fruit "shakes." *See* **Drinks** page 79.)

- **Berries.** A rich source of the phytochemicals *lycopene* and *ellagic acid*, both of which help prevent cell damage. Not to mention the abundance of antioxidant vitamins you'll find in blackberries, blueberries, boysenberries, cranberries, raspberries, and strawberries.

- **Citrus.** Though some nutritionists recommend reducing the acid in your system, especially when you have cancer, others disagree. In moderation, grapefruits, lemons, limes, oranges, and tangerines will offer benefit, because citrus fruits are known to be rich in almost 60 different plant chemicals that fight cancer.

- **Mangoes.** This powerhouse fruit is even higher in beta-carotene and other carotenoids than apricots, cantaloupe, or peaches—which should also be part of your diet.

- **Papayas.** Also full of beta-carotene, papaya is even richer in vitamin C—making it doubly strong as an immune booster.

- **Red grapes.** More often associated with heart-healthy diets, red grapes are high in antioxidants which cleanse the blood of free radicals. The skin also contains tartaric acid (as does the skin of raisins) which helps fight diseases and cancers of the colon.

Grains. Some grains can be a bit hard to digest. Others—particularly wheat—often trigger allergic reactions that can masquerade as indigestion or ulcerative problems. None are recommended as cancer fighters, but if you enjoy grains in your diet, the preferable ones are:

- **Barley.** Barley is as high in protein as meat. Because of its nutritional riches, people in some cultures actually live, thrive, work hard, and stay healthy on a diet that is barley based. It's more versatile than other grains, and can be eaten as a cooked cereal, mixed into soup, or baked into breads. For those who love the chewiness of grain, naturopaths recommend switching to barley among other things, because the phytochemicals in barley can prevent tumor growth.

- **Brown rice.** Whole-grain brown rice is rich in the antioxidant minerals *selenium* and *zinc,* and also the bone-building minerals *phosphorous* and *magnesium.* It's a great energy source because it's rich in B vitamins, and also because it falls in the middle of the glycemic index so it doesn't make blood-sugar levels spike and drop. High in fiber, it also cleanses the system. Some consider it a near-perfect complex carbohydrate.

- **Oats.** Another heart-healthy choice, oats—in the form of oatmeal—can benefit us in cancer resistance by reducing the level of bad cholesterol, which can feed tumors. Oats, like brown rice, are a source of steady energy.

- **Quinoa.** From the Andes, quinoa (*keen*-wah) has the highest protein of any grain (16 percent) and is also a complete protein, with an amino acid profile much like milk. It's rich in iron, for blood building, and in the B vitamins and vitamin E. Quinoa is very easy to digest, making its energy quickly available to the body. Black quinoa has a rich, nutty flavor. Either white or black varieties can be substituted for rice, millet, or couscous in cooking. The fact that quinoa places little stress on the digestive system and is a fast re-energizer offers indirect benefits to those determined to resist cancer. In any case, its general and considerable benefits in a healthy diet make it a valuable nutritional ally.

Vegetables. In the vegetable section of your grocer's produce department you'll find even more topflight ingredients for a cancer-resisting diet—in fact, a natural "pharmacy" of food medicines. However, you will want to greatly reduce, or cut, your intake of starchy vegetables such as potatoes, corn, and sweet potatoes.

Again, because there are thousands of phytochemicals that aid us in cancer resistance, what follows will not be your only vegetable choices—but they are your *best* choices:

℞

PROBIOTICS

∽

"Friendly bacteria" inhabit the human intestinal tract, helping with digestion, producing B vitamins, and killing disease-causing bacteria, which boost immunity. There are some 500 species of these bacteria, also known as "probiotics."

Unfortunately, antibiotics, chemotherapy, and other anti-cancer medicines can wipe out these allies. So can birth control pills and cortisone. So can plain old stress. Then we're left with a sort of "Trojan Horse" effect—that is, we're open to attack from the inside.

To maintain or restore a healthy level of probiotics during an illness or when taking medications, you can:

→ eat a diet rich in fruits, vegetable, whole grains, and foods with bacteria cultures, such as yogurt with live active cultures.

→ take probiotics, available in supplement form in health food stores.

If you decide to supplement: Buy capsules, because the process that produces probiotic caplets or pills can reduce potency. Buy the bottle with the most recent date *and* the greatest potency.

- **Asparagus.** The National Cancer Institute will tell you that asparagus is the food highest in *glutathione*, a powerful antioxidant naturally produced in the body...but often in short supply because of poor nutrition. Another substance in asparagus, *rutin*, is an antidote to radiation poisoning. And asparagus is high in all the antioxidant vitamins—A, C, and E—plus the B-complex vitamins and potassium and zinc.

- **Bell peppers.** These crunchy vegetables are rich in antioxidants; thus they give a quick boost to the immune system. While the orange, green, and yellow varieties are high in vitamins like C, red bell peppers hold *three times* as much C and *20 times* as much of the cancer-fighting beta-carotene.

- **Carrots.** A rich source of two major antioxidants, vitamin A and mixed carotenoids, carrots are also high in the B-complex vitamins, and coumarin—another phytochemical with anticancer properties. Some people enjoy raw carrots as a crunchy substitute for, say, potato chips at lunch. Unless you are eating several raw carrots a day, you may want to take a beta-carotene or a mixed-carotenoid supplement.

- **Cruciferous vegetables—bok choy, broccoli, cabbage, cauliflower, and kohlrabi.** The cruciferous vegetables contain *sulforaphane*, which helps the body's natural enzymes to fight off carcinogens and other toxins. It also helps prevent tumors from forming. Or if they have already formed, it helps prevent them from growing. A potent antioxidant in cruciferous vegetables, *lutein*, protects eyesight and combats respiratory, stomach, and colon cancers.

Note: Of the cabbages, red cabbage is the best choice because it contains *anthocyanins* which do double-duty against cancer—first, as antioxidants which cleanse the blood of free radicals; second, as substances that greatly inhibit the formation and growth of tumors. Of the other crucifers, broccoli is the more potent all-around vegetable in anticancer nutrition, but cauliflower is easier to digest—a very important point when dealing with a delicate stomach. Finally: *Vegetables from this family are best eaten raw or slightly cooked (steamed)—definitely not boiled to a limp death.*

- **Garlic (and onions).** These two "roses" of the garden contain *thiols*, which are among the most potent cancer-fighting agents in the plant kingdom. Thiols are sulfur-containing compounds that severely restrict the flow of blood to tumors. If eating garlic and/or onions is a problem for you—or those you live with—consider taking your garlic in the form of descented supplements.

- **Dark-green leafy vegetables—alaria, arame, dulse, hijiki, kombu, nori, sea palm, and wakame.** If you've never shopped in Asian or specialty grocery stores, you may never have heard of these delicious greens, all of which are rich in cancer-resisting phytochemicals. Their flavors range from mild and subtly sweet to spicy and "mustardy" to briny. You'll just have to try them and see which ones you like—or mix them for a great seaweed salad. (Did I forget to mention what these are?) They can used in salads, soups, mixed with a main course, and in stir-fries, and as greens on a sandwich.

The dark-green leafies are important to cancer resistance because they bind with carcinogenic heavy metals we absorb from the environment and eliminate them from the body. They also bind with radioactive substances and help eliminate them, preventing further damage to RNA and DNA.

- **Legumes—especially aduki, garbanzo, and hokaido beans.** Beans, in general, are rich in water-soluble fiber, which bonds with waste products in the body, preventing them from being reabsorbed and harming cells and tissues. The following varieties offer various cancer-resisting benefits:

  → **Adukis** (or Adzukis) are high in protein, low in fat. They have a tonic benefit for the kidneys, which are stressed during cancer treatment due to the many new substances passing through the body. Some research shows they may play a special role in preventing breast cancer. Adukis are also easier to assimilate than other beans. A larger variety, hokaidos, are also available.

  → **Garbanzos** (or chickpeas) have great tonic benefit for the stomach, spleen, and pancreas, organs usually overtaxed by the toxins passing through the body due to cancer and many of its treatments. (If you've only tasted canned chickpeas, try cooking fresh ones—they have a whole different flavor, and offer much better nutrition.)

Note: Adding mint to bean dishes can help reduce the discomfort of bloating.

- **Mushrooms—bolete, maitake, morel, reishi, and shiitake.** These particular mushrooms are important in cancer resistance because they absorb and eliminate toxins from the body. They are also known to inhibit the growth of tumors. While they are a delicious addition to your diet, you may not want to eat mushrooms in quantity every day. In that case you can still benefit from their therapeutic quality by taking mushroom extract in supplement form.

Your carbohydrate goal. In a generally healthy diet, you will want *40 percent* of your caloric intake to come from complex carbohydrates. Remember, you want to greatly reduce your intake of simple carbohydrates, which affect the production of insulin and other hormones, contributing to serious health problems. In creating a cancer-resisting diet, you will want *50 to 60 percent* of your daily food intake to come from complex carbohydrates, expecially those described above.

℞

THE NEW "HERBAL FOODS"

∽

From snack bar to soft drinks...food manufacturers are taking advantage of the public's interest in herbs and the health benefits they offer. But do those more expensive foods with herbs in them really offer us the benefits we're after?

Researchers—even those who otherwise recognize the health benefits of herbal supplements—say no. Consider this:

- You have to drink 40 or more bottles of a beverage containing St. John's Wort to get a therapeutic dose.

- At the opposite extreme, some snack bars containing herbal additives hold megadoses. So you have no idea how much of an herbal substance you're getting...and no indication of the side effects this dose can trigger...*and* no printed warning about medications or other herbs with which *these* herbs will interact negatively.

Bottom line: Put your money into herb *supplements*. You'll know the dosage you're getting. And always ask your physician, pharmacist, nutritionist, or naturopath if there are known side effects or negative interactions with other herbs or medications.

Fats

Our cultural hysteria about fat has left many of us greatly misinformed about this important dietary substance.

In general, we need some fat in our daily diets in order to make fat-soluble vitamins—like A, D, E, and K—do their work. Fat is also needed to trigger the production of many hormones. Contrary to popular opinion, a no-fat diet is *not* a good diet—it's a diet you would go on if you want to make yourself seriously ill or to do yourself in slowly.

However, certain fats are bad for our health in general, and they can actually aid in the formation of cancer and can feed tumors once they've started. These are the omega-6, or transfatty acids. In a cancer-resisting diet you'll want to eliminate these as much as possible. Other fats are very beneficial, not only for overall health but because they contain substances that help in natural cancer resistance. These are the omega-3 essential fatty acids (EFAs), and you'll need to use the right amount of these beneficial fats in your diet. (More on the "right amount" at the end of this section.)

What food choices can you make in order to get the beneficial fats you need for cancer resistance? Keeping in mind that you want to eliminate animal fats as much as possible, your best choices are:

- **Butters—"regular old...," nut, and seed.** It's confusing, isn't it? One day we're supposed to switch from regular old butter to margarine. Then we're supposed to switch back. Hopefully, this will make things somewhat clearer.

If your main concern is reducing or eliminating cholesterol from your diet because your levels are high and you're at risk of developing coronary diseases, *then* you should reduce or eliminate milkfat butter from your diet. *But...*if your main concern is cancer resistance, you don't want the load of oils used in margarine. In that case, *a little bit of butter is better.*

Nut butters—including almond butter, cashew butter, and natural peanut butter—are a generally healthier choice. Seed butters—like sesame or sunflower butter—are even better choices.

Remember: Use any butter sparingly. You only need *a little* fat—not a lot. Finally, even though soy was highly recommended earlier, in other food products, soy butter is *not* recommended because of its poor nutritional quality.

- **Culinary oils—coconut, flax, hemp, olive, palm, and sesame.** These oils are all high in omega-3 essential fatty acids. Their other importance in relation to cancer resistance is that they do not become toxic in our system like other oils widely used in our foods.

Olive oil is the oil most often recommended, especially the "extra virgin" variety. It is low in saturated fat, high in important EFAs, and is also known to support liver and gallbladder function. Sesame oil is the other topflight choice. Readily available in the average grocery store, sesame oil is high in the antioxidant vitamin E and has as much iron as liver. In addition, it's high in two important amino acids, making it a source of vegetable protein as well.

Flax and hemp oils are also great alternatives in cancer resistance, but their taste may be a bit strong for some. So consider them "next best" choices.

Coconut oil has received bad press because it's high in polyunsaturated fat—and so if you're using it as part of a cancer-resisting diet, use it sparingly…for flavoring…because it will boost your cholesterol level, as will palm oil. Consider these "third best" choices.

Avoid: Because you want to eliminate fats that become toxic in the body and also promote tumor growth, there are two popular oils you'll want to avoid. While canola oil has been widely touted as a healthy choice—because it does not increase cholesterol—it is highly refined and very low in omega-3 fatty acids, which means it soon becomes mildly toxic in the body. Corn oil, also highly processed and nutritionally valueless, is to be ignored. Soy oil tastes bitter, is hard to digest, and it raises toxicity in the body.

Your dietary fat goal: In a generally healthy diet, about *30 percent* of your total daily caloric intake should come from healthy fats such as those described above.

In a cancer-resisting diet, however, experts recommend that your fat intake should be *half* of that, or even less—about *10* to *15 percent*. This is because fats tend to support tumor growth. But you need not worry about this if you are choosing the best dietary fats.

They'll be working for you, aiding your other nutritional and supplemental cancer fighters.

Drinks

In the interest of a generally healthy diet, we should all be drinking more water and natural drinks. And we would do well to eliminate carbonated soft drinks and highly processed juices as much as possible, because they're loaded with empty calories and unhealthy corn sweeteners.

In terms of cancer resistance, these drinks are your best choices:

- **Almond milk.** Almond milk is a healthful and good-tasting alternative to cows' milk or soy milk. Containing a cyanide-like substance that is not toxic to anything in the body but tumors, almond milk is a delightfully thirst-quenching way to enjoy this benefit.

- **Barley-grass juice.** *This drink is one of the most potent of natural foods when it comes to cancer resistance.* A wide range of studies have demonstrated that when cancer cells are exposed to the nutrients in barley grass, tumor growth is inhibited and possibly reversed. Of the "green drinks," the juice of barley grass is the more alkaline, making it the more beneficial drink for an anticancer diet. Like its grain, barley grass is a great source of protein and is high in vitamin A. The enzymes it contains aid in digestion, and it also reduces toxins in the system. Though green drinks may take some getting used to, drinking even a small amount delivers great benefits.

- **Fruit shakes.** Let's say you've had enough fruit salad…fruit shakes are a great midmorning or midafternoon treat. They lift the spirit, give you a natural energy boost, and flood your system with antioxidants, enzymes, minerals, phytochemicals, vitamins—all immune boosting and cancer resisting. Using almond or soy milk will increase the health benefits of this great snack.

- **Green tea.** This is a favorite of health-conscious people everywhere. Studies show that green tea is rich in antioxidants and in substances that work at the cellular level to inhibit tumor growth. Black tea has similar benefits, though green tea is definitely richer in these natural medicines.

- **Natural fruit and vegetable juices.** As noted above, frozen concentrates and bottled juices (usually made from concentrates, so you're paying mostly for water and packaging) are usually loaded with corn sweeteners. Your choice should be the natural fruit and vegetable juices sold in health food stores and in refrigerated cases in some grocery stores, because they deliver the cancer-fighting phytochemicals and natural fiber you need.

- **Soy milk.** Soy milk contains about the same amount of protein as cows' milk, but it has one-third the fat, less calories, and zero cholesterol. Its benefit in cancer resistance is its easy digestibility, along with its richness in iron—15 times more than cows' milk—for the building of healthy red blood cells.

- **Water.** When taking medications or supplements....when undergoing chemo- or radiation therapies...or when we're under stress of any kind—physical, emotional, or spiritual—we *need* more water. Drinking water that's been purified is a great way to boost your electrolytes and cleanse toxins from the blood stream and the tissues. Adding lime, lemon, or an orange slice to a cool, tall one will add flavor and interest.

Avoid Alcohol. If you are on anticancer medications, or if you are taking natural supplements, or if you are relying on food medicines to help you resist cancer, consuming quantities of alcohol will work against you. This does not mean you cannot enjoy a few sips of beer or wine with dinner. But it does mean you should cut out consumption of harder alcoholic beverages entirely...and otherwise go very light.

Your fluid intake goal: In any healthy diet plan, it's recommended that we drink up to eight 8-ounce glasses of fluid a day, preferably one or more of those on the list above.

This is especially important when taking medications, supplements, or undergoing chemo- or radiation therapy.

Fasting and Detox Plans

Occasionally, fasting and "detoxifying" your system is a good idea for anyone wanting to support good health. Some people schedule monthly fast days and quarterly or semiannual "detox" periods.

Fasting gives your body a chance to rest from the normal…and pretty much endless…process of digestion. It's a good way to give your physical being a rest from producing all those enzymes, acids, and hormones required for digestion and the transfer of energy into the cells. Fasting, of course, simply requires cutting way back on your eating, or to do without food for a certain period of time—from skipping one meal to avoiding food (and/or liquids) for a day or more.

Detoxing requires not only cutting out or back on food, it involves taking natural substances—like certain herbs or teas—that are supposed to help cleanse the body. Some are geared toward cleansing the blood. Others cleanse the linings of the digestive tract, especially the small and large intestines, of food residue.

Fasting…for health reasons. A fast that eliminates all foods and fluids is not necessary. In fact, it takes only hours before your body switches into starvation mode and begins to dissolve healthy tissue to survive. A healthier form of fasting might be eliminating red meat or any meat for a period of time, particularly if you then introduce plant-source protein and foods high in natural fiber in their stead.

If you have cancer…a much healthier choice is to adopt a diet based on the foods discussed in this chapter. A total fast is not recommended because it will further stress your body. And you need the energy and food medicines a healthy diet will give you.

If you are fasting for spiritual purposes you should follow your own conscience, but consider a *"Daniel Fast"*—that is, eating fruits, vegetables, water, and natural juices for a short period of time. In any case, if you are a cancer patient you should inform your healthcare practitioner you are fasting.

Detoxing. Good detox plans can be found in many books available in natural health food stores. Magazines like *Natural Health* run articles about detoxing, offering step-by-step guidance. You can check these out at: www.naturalhealthmag.com.

However, as with fasting, it's best to use a detox plan under the guidance of a physician, nutritionist, or naturopath.

If you have cancer, it is essential to let your physician know what you are planning…to be sure that none of the herbs you'll be using react negatively with medicines you're taking.

It is never a good idea to stop drinking water and/or other healthy fluids when fasting or detoxing.

5

Physical Resilience

A ll of the techniques we've looked at so far—mental, spiritual, or dietary—have the benefit of building immunity and assisting in cancer resistance.

We can improve our ability to resist cancer even more if we add strategies to our health regimen that build better overall physical stamina and strength. These are what give us the physical resilience we need to maintain health and overcome disease.

Studies show that men and women who work out regularly build physical stamina, improve the quality of their sleep, and improve digestion, circulation, respiration, metabolism, and the elimination of toxins from their bodies. In addition, immune response rises sharply.

If you're interested in cancer resistance, I encourage you to do two things immediately:

First, if you don't have a regular workout schedule—*get into one!* Practically speaking, I realize that most of us have a very hard time carving two hours out of our daily schedule, three times a week, for a workout.

Also if you are facing cancer now and experiencing fatigue from the illness itself or as a result of medical therapies, you are not able to handle a strenuous workout. And in fact healthcare professionals recommend that people with cancer *not* engage in strenuous, over-taxing exercise routines. If you have cancer, you will only want to engage in light to moderate workouts.

Second, use the simpler strategies from this chapter to increase strength, mental clarity, emotional balance, and spiritual buoyancy.

These great strategies begin with the least strenuous, and move up to those that will give you a moderate workout. As you'll see, the overall-health and cancer-resistance benefits are terrific.

Strategies for Increasing Physical Resilience

Strategy #1: Breathe Deeply

One of the absolute basics of good health is good breathing. Believe it or not, there is a way to breathe that boosts overall wellness and immunity. Unfortunately, few of us breathe this way.

Much of the time our breathing is shallow. It's the kind of breathing we do when we're at rest or moving along at our normal pace. We use only about one-third of our lungs' capacity. Then there are times of stress or tension when our breathing becomes shallower still—as little as a quarter of the lungs' capacity. When we're under a lot of job, relationship, or health stress…or when we're down and depressed…we breathe shallowly much of the time.

Two physical problems result from shallow breathing. First, waste gases build up in our lungs, blood, body tissue, and cells. We feel achy, fatigued, even lethargic, unaware that these are physiological symptoms of the toxins and acids accumulating in the very fibers of our being. Second, we deprive our bodies of the oxygen needed at the most basic level of life—healthy cell reproduction.

On another level, shallow breathing leaves the muscle groups of our upper body feeling lethargic as metabolism slows. Stress breathing leaves our muscles tense. In both cases immune function drops.

To boost immunity and overall well-being, we need to practice deep breathing.

How to do it:

1. Notice how you're breathing right now.

Normally, we use only the chest muscles to inhale, filling just the top part of our lungs with air. Feel which muscles you are using.

2. Now use your diaphragm to help you inhale.

Your diaphragm is the big muscle below your rib cage. You'll know you're using your diaphragm to breathe because your belly will rise and fall, not just your chest. (This is the way babies breathe naturally. Sadly, it's a habit that shallow and stress breathing trains out of us.)

Note: Deep breathing is likely to make you light-headed unless you refine your technique. So…

3. Close your lips. Breathe in slowly through your nose.

To slow your inhalation, try breathing in to the count of *five*. Remember to use your stomach muscles. The point is to slowly fill your lungs to full capacity…and without holding your breath.

4. Relax your lips, as if you're blowing out a candle. Exhale through your mouth.

Don't exhale too quickly. Try it to the count of *three*.

5. Repeat the pattern for two minutes. Concentrate on your counting.

The goal is to keep up the pattern without becoming light-headed. You'll find that a two-minute "workout" is enough to begin with!

Benefits:

1. Oxygen is injected into the bloodstream. Here, it's used in building healthy new red blood and tissue cells and in fighting diseased cells. Cancer cells, in particular, hate oxygen. In addition, with more oxygen circulating to the brain, we experience greater mental clarity and alertness.

2. Circulation increases. Toxins are moved much more quickly out of the tissues and bloodstream. Nutrients move more efficiently to cells for healthy reproduction.

3. Muscles throughout the whole upper body release stored physical tension. The overall calm triggers the deep-relaxation response. Emotional calm returns. In addition...

4. Deep relaxation boosts immunity by increasing the production of disease-resisting hormones, T-cells, and macrophages.

Deep breathing is the simplest of the physical resistance-building strategies. It can be done anywhere, even if you're confined to bed or riding in a vehicle. Likewise, anyone can do this, even if you suffer from respiratory conditions, like asthma or allergies.

Many people use deep breathing together with meditation or contemplation and find that it sharpens mental and spiritual focus.

Strategy #2: Stretch for It

When we're feeling stiff or fatigued, it's because natural acids, like lactic acid, have built up in our muscle tissues. Circulation and metabolism are low. Toxins are building. Immune resistance is down.

If we have a disease like cancer, the body will produce even more toxins than normal. These additional poisons will be stored up in our tissues unless they're expelled. Add to that the toxins that build as anticancer medications break down, or the toxins created by radiation or chemotherapy.

Put this all together, and you'll see why it's so important to use stretching as a strategy in disease resistance.

How to do it:

Sitting on the floor is recommended, but if that's uncomfortable, sit on a bed or in a chair.

1. Pick an open space on the floor. Sit with your legs comfortably apart.

All your movements must be slow and gentle. Never force tight muscles or sore joints. The goal is to express lactic acid and other natural wastes that have built up. Repeat each step that follows, until the muscle group being worked relaxes.

Remember to use cleansing breaths between stretches.

2. Begin with your neck.

Holding up that 8 1/2-pound bowling ball we call a head is a lot of work! But never stretch neck muscles by rolling your head, as that can cause serious damage to the small delicate disks and vertebrae in your neck.

Turn your head slightly to the right, and slowly drop your chin until it touches your collarbone. Return to starting position. Repeat on the left side. This stretches the group of small muscles that run from the base of the skull to the shoulder blade.

3. Stretch your upper back.

Raise your left shoulder slowly toward your left ear. At the same time, push your shoulder forward, until you can feel the back muscles between your shoulder blade and spine stretch. Return to starting position. Do the same thing, using the right shoulder.

4. Chest and abdominals.

Extend your arms in front and lay one hand on the other, palms down. Slowly raise your arms straight over your head, allowing your diaphragm to expand as you inhale. As you reach toward the sky, allow your chest and abdominal muscles to stretch.

Still stretching, use your right hand to gently draw your left arm across and in front of your face. Feel the muscles down the back side of your left ribs stretch. Repeat for the benefit of your right side.

Now, using your right hand, gently draw your left arm across and *behind* your head. Feel the muscles in your shoulder and down the side of your left ribs stretch. Repeat, right.

The tendency when stretching is to hold your breath. Keep breathing!

5. Back-of-the-leg muscles.

(This can be done standing, or seated with legs out straight.) With your arms outstretched, hands one over the other, slowly bend at the waist and reach for your left foot. Keep your left leg straight. Don't bend your knee…and *don't force.* Feel the buttock and hamstring muscles stretch. Repeat to make the right side happy.

6. Quadriceps and calf muscles.

(From a seated position or lying down.) Point your left foot as straight out as you can. Feel the muscles all the way up the front of your leg stretch. Hold for a moment, then relax. Repeat on the right.

Now push out the heel of your left foot. Feel your calf muscles stretch. Repeat with the right.

7. Buttocks and quadriceps.

(Seated or lying down.) Bend your left leg and clasp the knee with both hands. Slowly draw your knee up to your chest as far as you can. Feel the buttocks and quadriceps stretch. Relax. Repeat on the other side.

Benefits:

1. Cardiovascular functioning—heart rate and blood flow—is increased.

2. Oxygen is delivered more rapidly to the cells, along with nutrients for the creation of healthy new tissue and red blood cells.

3. Toxins are carried away from tissues more quickly, for rapid elimination.

4. Stress is released, physically, mentally, and spiritually.

The slow, deliberate *flexing* and *extension* of our large muscle groups is a gift we can give to our body. It's an excellent way to start or end the day because it energizes in the morning and relaxes at night. A modified stretching workout can also be done at work, on a plane or train, or in a car.

Variation: Yoga is a wonderful exercise regimen that has helped people for some 8,000 years. Along with stretching your large-muscle groups, it builds muscle strength in a natural way. You can easily find yoga instruction in classes, books, and videos, that offer you the benefits of a light to moderate workout.

If you are a person with strong spiritual convictions that are not Eastern, don't worry. You will find many instructors who do not push you to adopt philosophies or religious beliefs, so you can enjoy the health benefits of a yoga workout.

Strategy #3: Massage Therapy

Disease resistance requires our muscles to be loose and not storing acids and tensions. Sometimes stretching is not enough, and our muscles need additional help.

In some cultures, massage therapy has been widely accepted for centuries as an important aspect of a good-health regimen. Here in the West, we are just discovering its benefits.

Massage therapy involves the simple manipulation of muscles, using rubbing, warmth, and pressure.

If you're like most people, you may feel uneasy at first being touched by a stranger. Give yourself time to get over it. You'll be amazed at how great it feels to relax under the care of an expert.

How to do it:

For simple massage therapy, make an appointment with a licensed massage therapist (LMT), or use one of the many books on massage now available on the market and work with a partner at home.

To find an LMT in your area, call the American Massage Therapy Association at (847) 864-0123. You may also be able to get this information from your physician or therapist, or from your county or city mental health department.

Benefits:

1. Circulation is increased. Toxins are more quickly moved out of the body.

2. Physical, emotional, and spiritual stress is released. The deep-relaxation response is triggered, boosting the whole immune system.

Strategy #4: An Immunity-Boosting Walk

Walking at even a *moderate* pace is a great way to improve disease resistance by improving respiration and increasing physical stamina. Add to your daily walk a mental strategy like "Opening the Mental Pressure Valve" (see chapter 2) or a spiritual practice like "Flow Praying" (chapter 3), and you will also find yourself gaining a healthier frame of mind and a wiser perspective on life.

Sure, almost *anybody* can walk. But there are things you can do to make for a truly *great* walk, one that boosts your immunity and overall health.

How to do it:

1. Choose two or three routes.

Try to pick a short route (10-minute walk), a midrange route (20-minute walk), and a long course (30 minutes or more). This will give you changes of scenery and options to choose from, depending on how much time or energy you have to walk on any given day. Include at least one indoor "route"—say, inside a local shopping mall—to use during bad weather.

2. Don't go "cheap" on the footwear.

The $15 discount house "cheapies" are poorly made. Your feet and legs need better support. You don't need to spend a lot of money to get better-made walking shoes. This means shoes that "breathe" because they're made of fabric (not leather) uppers...and that also support your instep and ankle well.

3. Get your walking rhythm and your pulse up.

You'll want to achieve a rhythm to your stride that is aggressive enough to encourage proper deep breathing and that you can sustain through most of your walk. You can easily check your pulse by placing the index and middle finger of your left hand on your right medial artery—that blue "pencil" line at the base of the left thumb.

Target Heart-Rate Range

On the next page are target heart rates you'll want to reach if you'd like to get a good aerobic workout during your walk (or any other exercise). Achieving your target rate for at least 30 minutes, three times a week, is very beneficial.

Age	Range
25	120 to 156 beats per minute *(20 to 26 beats per 10 seconds)*
35	114 to 150 beats per minute *(19 to 25 beats per 10 seconds)*
45	108 to 138 beats per minute *(18 to 23 beats per 10 seconds)*
55	102 to 132 beats per minute *(17 to 22 beats per 10 seconds)*
65	96 to 126 beats per minute *(16 to 21 beats per 10 seconds)*

4. Let your mind and spirit relax.

Walking, while relaxing all mental and spiritual stress away is a great way to unburden your physical being of these stresses.

This is also an excellent time to pray, unburdening your soul to God…or if you prefer, meditate on a *positive affirmation* from sacred Scriptures or inspirational writing.

5. At the end of your walk, give yourself a good 10- to 15-minute cool-down period.

After elevating your heart rate, it's not a good idea to sit or lie down immediately. Give your heart rate a chance to return to normal.

Benefits:

1. Respiration increases. Better-oygenated blood reaches healthy cells and muscle tissues. Cancerous cells are inhibited by the increased oxygen.

2. Circulation increases, and the muscles are "worked-out." Nutrients are moved more quickly to the cells. Toxins are more swiftly removed from the body.

Strategy #5: Nonimpact Aerobics

Nonimpact Aerobics (NIA) offer a great workout experience...without the pounding intensity of normal aerobics. It's a great way to exercise if your energy level is down but you want more than stretching or deep breathing.

NIA is a blend of stretching, fluid motion, *and* proper breathing. The routines are comprised of slower, more graceful movements—but the concentration on "right form" adds the benefits of muscle toning and elevated respiration and circulation.

NIA was developed by two aerobics instructors, Debbie and Carlos Rosas, who discovered that high-impact aerobics often cause serious injuries for those who jump into those challenging routines without good prior conditioning, and also for people with health conditions.

How to do it:

1. Check local community centers, gyms, and health clubs to sign up for NIA classes.

2. Purchase a videotaped version of a NIA workout. These are available in many larger bookstores and through on-line book and tape dealers.

Benefits:

1. Metabolism is increased. We experience better appetite and digestion.

2. Respiration and heart rate increase. More oxygen and nutrients reach the cells.

3. Brain chemistry achieves a higher state of functioning. The neurotransmitter chemicals that create better moods are produced, giving us a mental lift.

4. Muscle strength is increased. We experience more endurance and resilience.

Final thought: If it will help you to stick to a workout plan, find a buddy to try these routines with you.

6

Natural Supplements

Some of the natural supplements discussed in this chapter are known to cause negative reactions in the body when taken in combination with prescription medications. Some are also known to cause negative reactions when taken in combination with other supplements. When a supplement is known to react negatively in combination, or when specific cautions are known, this is noted.

Be advised: Scientific testing of natural supplements is still ongoing. Therefore, it is not possible at this time to list all the possible contraindications that may occur after taking natural supplements.

When adding natural supplements to a cancer-resistance plan you should do so in consultation with a healthcare professional.

Always notify your physician and/or pharmacist if you are using supplements.

Now that you've been sobered by reading the above cautions—here are some other cautions to consider, lest you give in to the temptation to skip this chapter.

First, many pharmaceutical drugs inhibit the body's use of vitamins and minerals, interrupting digestion and the absorption of nutrients and also the production of hormones. The list includes not only anticancer medications but such common drugs as antibiotics and birth control pills. Even over-the-counter "drugs," like antacids and aspirin, can prevent the body from absorbing important micronutrients from our food.

Many natural supplements provide a tonic effect that boosts the whole body. Others assist in healthy digestion and the assimilation of nutrients from our diet.

Second, pharmaceutical drugs—especially those used to fight cancer—have harsh side effects. Their job is to attack cancer, and they are toxic. Unfortunately, as they combat cancer, they also work against healthy organs and the proper functioning of the body's many systems.

Natural supplements that combat cancer are, generally, much gentler in the way they affect the processes that lead to cancer and the ones that occur once cancer has started. Certain supplements also help safeguard the organs from the toxic effects of chemo- and radiation therapies.

The bottom line is: Natural supplements most definitely do offer many benefits when used as part of a cancer-resistance plan.

Add to these thoughts this final comment, on a separate but related matter: Every one of us needs a healthy diet that gives us the balance of nutrients to keep our bodies' various systems running well. The problem is, very few of us eat a well-balanced diet. Not only that, but in the course of processing, the foods we eat are often depleted of many of their nutrients.

For these reasons, supplementation is a good idea for all of us.

Doctors

Despite the growing body of evidence (even scientific studies) supporting the effectiveness of natural supplements, some medical doctors are still against the use of supplements in preventing or treating cancer. These are the doctors who will tell you supplements are pretty much a waste of your money. Many other physicians are indifferent, or think the therapeutic benefits are overstated. There are, actually, good reasons why this mind-set exists.

First, many of the claims made about "natural cancer cures" are anecdotal (based on hearsay). They are not supported—or at least, not yet supported—by the kind of long-range scientific studies the medical community relies on. In the case of many natural supplements, studies are only just now underway, and it will be years more before anything but preliminary findings are published. This is because the use of a substance must be tracked in a set population, under controlled circumstances, over a long time. This is very important in observing not only true effectiveness, but possible damaging side effects that may not show up right away. If there are negative effects of taking high doses of certain natural substances, they might not show up for *years*…especially given the fact that herbs are slow-acting. Which leads to the second point.

Some natural substances—herbs, as a case in point—*do* take longer to work. Their potency is cumulative. In dealing with an aggressive disease like cancer, time is very much of the essence. Aggressive courses of chemotherapy and/or radiation therapy *and* quick surgery are often needed.

Third, the manufacture of natural supplements is not regulated by the U.S. FDA (as of this writing). Some laboratory tests have shown that a capsule of a given substance is actually mostly filler and contains little or none of the substance it is supposed to be carrying. Doctors point out that for any substance to be therapeutically effective, it is very important that it be delivered to the body in consistent doses. Some today, less tomorrow, none the day after is not effective.

Fourth, fantastic claims some manufacturers have made about the "cancer-walloping punch" of certain natural supplements have put healthcare professionals…and savvy healthcare consumers…on guard. We are right to be skeptical about claims that any single product can "improve sex drive, regrow hair, *and* is also the cancer cure that physicians and pharmaceutical companies don't want you to know about."

Be Knowledgeable

Nonetheless, more and more evidence is amassing—from cancer survivors and laboratory testing—that indicate natural supplements are beneficial in building cancer resistance.

As a result, attitudes in the medical community are changing, and you may wish to locate a physician who is supportive of your plan to use natural supplements to help resist cancer.

Once again, though, it's in your best interest to become well informed about the specific natural supplements you want to try. Learn what they do and how to use them. Be aware of any cautions you need to exercise.

In general, you should know these things:

Some natural supplements will interfere with the body's use of pharmaceuticals. Some will react negatively with drugs—in effect, poisoning your system. Possibly the ones you're planning to use. In the lists that follow, some cautions are listed. Check with your physician and pharmacist for the most up-to-date information and studies.

Before you begin a course of natural supplements, *always* discuss your plans with your physician. It is absolutely essential that he or she know what supplements are active in your system when working with you on a treatment plan.

Check up on the companies from whom you buy your supplements. There is information in this chapter that will help you do this. You may also be able to do this through your local, natural health food store.

Finally, there are no "magic bullets" when it comes to preventing or treating cancer with natural supplements. If claims sound too good to be true, they probably are. A balanced, whole-person approach to health or recovery *is* the best approach.

Cancer-Resistance Benefits of Natural Supplements

What follows are lists of natural supplements most often recommended to aid in cancer resistance. They are recommended for their ability to benefit us in one or more of the biological processes that lead to cancer, or to help reverse an unhealthy process once cancer has begun, including:

➔ assisting in the reproduction of healthy DNA and RNA and the creation of new cells

➔ removing damaged cells (free radicals) from the body before they cause damage to still-healthy cells, veins, and tissues

➔ having a "tonic" effect on the whole body—boosting respiration, circulation, elimination, and promoting greater wellness overall

➔ hindering the growth of tumors

➔ promoting the development of healthy red blood cells, important because of cancer's dislike of oxygen

→ strengthening immune response by helping in the creation of T-cells and macrophages—those "soldier cells" that attack intruders within the body

→ protecting the liver, kidneys, and other organs from the toxins produced by tumors and/or the negative effects of chemotherapy drugs or radiation

Make sure to read the very important section on "How to Take Supplements" at the close of this chapter.

A Small Apothecary
of Natural Cancer-Resisting Supplements
∽∽∽

The Amino Acid Shelf

- *N-Acetylcysteine (NAC).* Glutathione is an enzyme our bodies produce and a naturally occurring antioxidant. It protects against free radicals and toxins, the ones produced by tumors as well as those resulting from radiation or chemotherapy. So it can help prevent or cure cancer *and* can be used to reboost the immune system during aggressive medical therapies. However, glutathione itself is poorly absorbed when taken orally.

  NAC, taken orally, converts to glutathione once it is absorbed into our cells. There it enhances the reproduction of healthy DNA. By supporting liver function, it also blocks the toxic effect of various chemotherapy drugs and combats toxins created by tumors. NAC is sometimes sold in combination with coenzyme Q-10.

  Cautions: *Healthy people should not use NAC supplements. Doing so can be very harmful.* NAC supplementation can be beneficial only to people whose blood has been tested and shown to be low in glutathione. (Under normal conditions, only people with tumors will register low levels of glutathione.)

  If you are being treated with chemotherapy, you should consult with your physician before supplementing with NAC.

- *SAM-e.* This substance is being widely used in the treatment of depression. But its benefits in cancer resistance are acknowledged as well.

SAM-e (S-adenosylmethionine) is the amino acid most needed for the repair of DNA.

Therefore it is essential to healthy cell reproduction and growth. Though it is a naturally occurring amino acid many factors can hinder its production in the body—including aging and a diet too high in animal protein. SAM-e also stimulates many immune functions, making it a valuable anti-cancer agent.

℞

QUALITY SUPPLEMENTS—HOW CAN YOU KNOW?

∿

News and stories abound about laboratories that have tested natural supplements…only to discover that the substance named on the jar's label doesn't even exist in some of the capsules. Or that the quality and potency of the substance varies widely from one manufacturer's lot to the next.

If you are going to make natural supplements part of something as important as a cancer-resistance plan…how can you have greater assurance that the supplements you're taking are actually high in quality?

Here are two ways you can check out the supplement manufacturers you're buying from:

Dietary Supplement Quality Initiative. DSQI reviews natural supplements and makes its findings available to the public. Read up on the latest supplement news at their website: www.dsqi.org. If you cannot find a review of the supplement(s) you are researching, you may wish to call them at: (617) 734-4123.

ConsumerLab.com. This website posts the findings of dozens of independent labs that buy supplements off-the-shelf, just like you do, and tests them. They test for purity, the accuracy of information on the label, and consistency. Candid test results are free to you by just logging on.

The Food Extract Shelf

- *Bilberry extract.* Bilberries are the greatest source of certain antioxidants, known as *anthocyanins* and *proanthocyanins.* These substances, besides eliminating free radicals in the blood, may also help to hold the growth of tumors in check. (See p. 70 for a previous discussion of antioxidants.)

A WORD ABOUT ANTIOXIDANTS
∼

Because you are going to be reading a lot in this chapter about antioxidants you should know, if you don't already, what they are and their importance in the physiological process they affect. In the normal process of living and aging, cells wear out, and at the same time genes break down in the course of reproduction. This process of biological "oxidation" has been likened to the rusting, or corrosion, of metal. It is because of this process that damaged cells, or free radicals are formed and cancer is likely to occur. Antioxidants are substances that bond with free radicals, preventing them from damaging still-healthy cells, until they are eliminated from the body.

- *Bromelain.* This enzyme, extracted from the stems of pineapples, is used in treating disorders and diseases in which inflammation occurs. As a support in cancer treatment, it may be used to calm secondary inflammations naturally, allowing the immune system to refocus its energies on the primary problem—cancer. It may also inhibit the flow of blood to tumors, helping to prevent their rapid growth.

- *Carotenoids.* Carotenoids are phytochemicals, compounds found in plants that promote our resistance to substances not found in the natural environment such as chemicals and other potential carcinogens. Until recently, it was thought that beta-carotene, one of hundreds of carotenoids, was *the* effective anticancer member of this family of antioxidants. Recent studies have caused experts to be less sure about beta-carotene's specific importance. And so the current recommendation is to supplement with the mixed carotenoids for cancer protection.

Caution: You should not smoke—ever—let alone when you have cancer. But if you do smoke, you should get your beta-carotene from foods and not from supplements. Some studies indicate synthetic beta-carotene may increase the risk of lung cancer for smokers.

- *Fish oil (omega-3 fatty acids.)* Cancer researchers have suggested that a diet made up of 15 to 20 percent healthy fats will help with both the prevention and treatment of cancer. Research shows tumor growth is promoted by taking in too many "bad fats"—that is, the omega-6 fatty acids found in most animal fat and also in certain vegetable oils. Omega-3 fatty acids, the healthy fats, are readily available to us in fish oils and certain plant oils, and they appear to help prevent the spread of cancer.

  Fish oil is the most recommended of the omega-3s, because it's rich in eicosapentaenoic acid (EPA), a cancer-fighting form of fat. If you are a vegetarian, you may wish to supplement with flaxseed oil, another source of EPA.

- *Modified citrus pectin (MCP).* Cancer moves from one cell to another by interactions that occur as the membrane of a cancerous cell stimulates the cells next to it to also become cancerous. Derived from citrus fruit fiber, MCP is known to interfere with this cell-to-cell transmission of cancer. MCP appears to interrupt the transmission—in medical terms, it seems to keep cancer from metastasizing—because it contains *rhamnogalacturonon,* a substance that supports the body's tumor fighting T-cells.

- *Grapeseed extract.* This extract contains anthocyanin, a bioflavonoid and antioxidant that scours the bloodstream in search of free radicals. It is most effective when taken in combination with vitamin C. (*See* Bioflavonoids.) The effectiveness of grapeseed extract as an antioxidant is also known to be several times greater than vitamins C and E and beta-carotene.

Caution: If you are taking blood thinners, or if you are pregnant or trying to conceive, you should consult your physician before using grapeseed extract.

- *Green tea.* Green tea is an effective whole-body tonic that stimulates the immune system, making it one of the simplest (and enjoyable!) cancer-resistance "treatments" you can add to your daily regimen.

  As a natural cancer treatment, green tea also contains the bioflavanoid *quercitin.* Studies have shown that quercitin can help weaken malignant cells, making them more responsive to chemotherapy and other treatments.

- *Cartilage.* Harvested from sharks and cows, the cancer-resistance benefits of cartilage supplementation comes from a protein that may inhibit blood flow to tumors. Some controversy surrounds the use of cartilage in cancer-resistance therapy, since most evidence to support claims of its effectiveness comes from anecdote rather than conclusive scientific study.

- *Curcumin.* This plant extract sits on our shelves at home under labels marked "Turmeric" and "Curry Powder." Curcumin is an antioxidant that affects each stage of a cancer's development, making it an important addition to a natural cancer-resistance plan.

  First, curcumin's ability to protect healthy DNA is greater than other, more commonly used antioxidants. Second, it eliminates mutagens—chemical substances that cause cell mutation. Finally, it reduces inflammations, which cause the body to produce hormones that can support tumor growth once it's begun. Curcumin is available in therapeutic doses in capsule form, usually in combination with certain vitamins and/or herbs.

- *Garlic.* Certain sulfur-containing compounds in garlic, known as thiols, have shown to be highly effective in reducing the growth of new blood cells around and in tumors, inhibiting their growth.

- *Ginger.* Ginger is widely used to ease nausea, but its possible benefits in cancer resistance have not been known until recently. Compounds in ginger, known as *phenols,* are thought to be responsible for prohibiting the development of certain cancers—in particular, skin cancer.

- *Maitake mushrooms.* A substance in the maitake mushroom, *beta glucan,* activates killer T-cells and macrophage cells, both of which are potent cancer fighters. This substance, sold in powdered, extracted form, acts as a whole-body tonic and stimulates the entire immune system's responsiveness. Cancer patients who are undergoing chemotherapy and who supplement with maitake extract often experience other great side benefits, including a decrease in nausea and vomiting and the ability to retain a healthy appetite, which add up to an increase in vital energy.

- *Reishi mushrooms.* These mushrooms have been used for centuries in oriental medicine.

  As a cancer preventative, the powerful antioxidants in reishis act as a whole-body tonic, boosting the immune system. Other compounds in reishis stimulate the healthy duplication of RNA and DNA within the cells. As a detoxifier, other reishi compounds help protect the liver from the damaging effects of toxins.

The Herb Shelf

- *Aloe vera.* Derived from the leaves of the aloe plant, the extract—aloe vera—has been used successfully by gastroenterologists and practitioners of natural medicine in the treatment of inflammatory bowel conditions, including ulcerative colitis and Crohn's Disease. It is a natural laxative, and its compounds promote the healing of inflammation.

There is also evidence of its ability to promote cellular health when the intestinal lining has experienced severe irritation and damage. Therefore, it may be beneficial in the prevention of cancer for those who are at higher risk because of such intestinal disorders.

Caution: Aloe vera, when used as a laxative, can cause severe cramping. For this reason it is not recommended for use during pregnancy. If you want to use aloe vera for this or any other purpose—especially during an intestinal flare-up or if you have cancer—consult with your healthcare professional first.

- *Amalaki (Indian gooseberry).* The extract of this fruit from an Asian tree is highly regarded in Oriental medicines as a supertonic. Because it's known to stimulate the production of healthy red blood cells and promote healthy tissue growth, it's also recommended by many practitioners of natural medicine for use in cancer resistance.

- *Astragalus.* Astragalus is a Chinese herb known to stimulate the production of T-cells. It's even more effective in stimulating immune response when used in combination with Siberian ginseng.

  Astragalus seems to greatly enhance the effectiveness of *interleukin-2.* Consult with your physician about this. Physicians may recommend the use of a drug that is actually derived from astragalus, which makes it possible to measure the therapeutic dose. But commercially produced extracts of astragalus are also available directly to you.

- *Burdock (Gobo).* This common weed has been used in folk medicine for centuries as a "purifier." Burdock contains *inulin,* a compound which stimulates the production of white blood cells, thus increasing our defenses against cancer-causing invaders. It also stimulates liver function, helping with blood purification. And it is a mild diuretic, once again helping to detoxify the body. It's sometimes sold in fresh, root form under its Asian name, Gobo.

- *Cat's Claw (Una de Gato).* Herbs with names like "Cat's Claw" can trigger skepticism in even the most cooperative medical doctor. Even more so when it's told that this one comes from the Peruvian rainforest. Nonetheless, it has demonstrated its potency as an antitumor and immunity-enhancing substance in folk medicine…and now, under the scrutiny of Western scientific study. Certain compounds in Cat's Claw scavenge for free radicals, while others have anti-inflammatory and antitumor properties.

  Cautions: This herb appears to be nontoxic for most people in general. However, it should not be taken during pregnancy, or if you are taking antiulcer medications, or if you have received an organ transplant. You should consult with your physician before taking Cat's Claw.

- *Chapparal.* This is another herb that comes with strong cautions. Chapparal has been highly recommended for years because of its powerful antioxidant properties, and many practitioners of natural medicine urge its use in preventing and fighting cancer.

  Caution: Do not use this herb if you have liver or kidney disease. All others should use it only under the guidance of a qualified herbalist and/or naturopathic doctor with a specific knowledge of herbs. Notify your physician if you are taking Chapparal.

- *Echinacea.* Following on the heels of the last two recommendations…echinacea is now so widely recommended for so many things, it may seem fairly lightweight as a cancer-resisting herb.

  Echanacea purpurea, one of several echinacea species sold, is the one you want. Preliminary studies have shown *this* type of echinacea to be an effective combative agent against the formation of new cells in tumors. In addition, it boosts the immune system by promoting the development of macrophages, which scour damaged cells and other debris traveling in the bloodstream. Finally, it can help reduce the chances of colds, viruses, and secondary infections that opportunistically take hold in someone weakened by cancer.

- *Milk thistle.* The active ingredient in milk thistle, *silymarin,* protects the body from the negative effects of many traditional cancer therapies. On a biochemical level, it helps prevent the depletion of glutathione. (*See* N-Acetylcysteine.) The major benefit of milk thistle supplementation, perhaps, is that silymarin protects the liver and kidneys from toxins. Along with that, it works within the liver to help regenerate healthy tissue, making it a supplement that's very useful in conjunction with traditional medical approaches when treating liver cancer.

The Hormone Shelf

- *Melatonin.* Produced by the pineal gland in the brain, melatonin is nature's sleeping pill. As darkness descends, melatonin is increased...until we drowse into sleep. Supplementation with melatonin can help restore natural and deep sleep when worry, pain, or restlessness associated with illness interrupt it—and good sleep is necessary to keep the immune system working. Melatonin also directly stimulates the part of our immune system that inhibits tumor growth.

  Melatonin is sometimes used in therapeutic treatment plans in combination with interleukin-2, which can be ineffective when used on its own. You may wish to discuss this with your doctor if interleukin-2 treatment is planned.

The Mineral Shelf

- *Calcium and Magnesium.* These two minerals, taken in combination, offer many health benefits—from boosting brain power, to strengthening bones, to boosting energy, to maintaining healthy heart and nerve function. Add to those: anti-cancer benefits.

- *Selenium.* Selenium is an effective antioxidant trace mineral. Combined with vitamin C and E, or with one of the other powerful antioxidants, it can have great therapeutic value in the early stages of cancer to prevent metastasis, especially when taken in dosages higher than the U.S. FDA's recommended daily dosages. It also breaks down toxic chemicals in the body, such as carcinogens we absorb from the environment and toxins produced by tumors.

  Caution: Though high doses of selenium can be tolerated, you must be carefully monitored by a physician to prevent toxicity.

- *Zinc.* This trace mineral stimulates healthy cell formation. For that reason it helps govern the reproduction of our genes. It's important to take zinc in combination with the trace mineral copper.

The Vitamin Shelf:

- *Vitamin A.* Vitamin A is one of the most potent of the antioxidants—the substances which bond with free radicals in the blood preventing cell damage and the wear and tear of blood vessels. For this reason, A is highly important to cancer resistance.

  Caution: Unlike most other vitamins, vitamin A is not water soluble, which means it can be stored and build up in the body's fat tissues. High doses, taken in a short period of time, can have a toxic effect. Follow manufacturer's directions carefully.

- *Vitamin B-Complex.* A wide range of important body functions are affected by this family of vitamins. They are quickly depleted when we are under physical, mental, or spiritual stress. All of the B vitamins, taken together, have an overall tonic effect, boosting energy by helping our bodies to use food fuel efficiently. One of the B vitamins, folic acid (known also as *folacin* or *folate*), works at the cellular level to repair and maintain damaged genes. B_6 *pyridoxene*, is known to empower the immune system. It helps in the production of new and healthy red blood cells and the creation of antibodies which fight disease.

- *Vitamin C.* This familiar vitamin is another of the antioxidants. As a cancer resistant, vitamin C is sometimes taken in doses higher than a manufacturer's or the U.S. FDA's recommended dosages. It has been shown to enhance the positive effects of most chemotherapy drugs.

  Certain claims have been made about the health and anti-cancer benefits of taking C in extremely high doses—up to100,000 milligrams per day, or *10 times* the maximum recommended dose. You can experience the therapeutic value of vitamin C by taking smaller doses than that, say, two or three times the recommended daily dose.

  Caution: Higher doses of vitamin C may cause cramping and diarrhea. Though not toxic, this is obviously not healthy or pleasant. If you experience this distress due to an intake of vitamin C that is too high for your system to tolerate, reduce the dosage you are taking immediately. Be sure to replenish your electrolytes with an increased intake of fluids, preferably water.

- *Bioflavonoids (vitamin P).* These water-soluble antioxidants greatly enhance the body's absorption and use of vitamin C. For this reason, they are often sold in combination. Derived from fruit and vegetable sources, bioflavonoids include *citrin, flavones, flavonols, hesperidin, quercetin, and rutin*—and now, when you see them on a label, you'll recognize these unfamiliar names and know what benefit these substances hold for you.

- *Coenzyme Q-10.* "CoQ-10" is a fat-soluble enzyme often found mixed in with vitamins on the shelves of pharmacies and health food stores. This enzyme is naturally produced in both plant and animal cells, where its primary job is to help cells derive energy from nutrients. Helping our cells get the most energy from passing nutrients is a great benefit when fighting an illness and the fatigue it causes. For this reason, it's very important in restoring vitality.

CoQ-10 is also a naturally occurring antioxidant. It works in combination with vitamin E to prevent vascular damage caused by free radicals. Often, however, environmental factors, illness, and even stress prevent our bodies from producing it in the quantities we need. Thus it is important to supplement.

If you have cancer and want to supplement with CoQ-10, you may wish to purchase it from manufacturers who combine it with *catalase* and *superoxide dimutase*—which are two other natural, antioxidant enzymes that are depleted during illness. Finally, although CoQ-10 is fat soluble, it's taken in small doses, greatly reducing the risk of buildup in the tissues and toxicity.

Caution: Consult with your physician before taking CoQ-10 if you are taking heart medications, as it may react negatively with some of these pharmaceuticals.

- *Vitamin D.* Recent clinical studies have shown that this vitamin may slow certain cancers, most notably breast and colon cancer.

- *Vitamin E.* Yet another important antioxidant, vitamin E has been tested and shown to block the formation of *nitrosamines,* chemical compounds we are sometimes exposed to that are known to cause cancer in animal experimentation. By blocking these damaging foreign compounds absorbed from the environment, E protects cell membranes. Studies indicate that E may reduce the risk of particular cancers, especially those that attack the lungs and liver.

How to Take Supplements

The answer is…just *take* them, right? Not so. You need some knowledge about how to take supplements—important knowledge:

Buy quality. Price is not an indicator of quality. Go to websites and organizations that test and rate natural supplements, and check out the manufacturer from whom you're buying. (*See above*: "Quality Supplements—How Can You Know?")

Read labels carefully. Some supplements must be taken with food. Others are more effective if taken in several doses over the course of a day. Many manufacturers will also list drugs and other supplements with which this particular substance will react negatively. This can hardly be emphasized enough: *Read the label.*

Increase your water intake. It is very important to increase your intake of fluids—preferably water—when taking supplements. This means taking in more than the few sips it requires to get the supplements down.

Increasing your water intake is important because many supplements make your liver and kidneys work harder, and water will help these vital organs do their work better and keep them functioning in a healthy manner. In some cases, you may be taking doses that are several times greater than the normally recommended daily dose, and so your liver and kidneys most definitely need the added help of more water.

Especially if you are on a regimen of cancer-resisting supplements (and medications) you should increase your water intake. Drink a minimum of four 8-ounce glasses of water a day, and build up to eight. Cool water, *not cold,* is best.

When taking herbs, more is not better. Certain supplements, like vitamins and minerals, do increase in effectiveness if you increase the daily dosage. It does not work the same way with herbs. Herbs are effective and build up potency over time. Upping the dose is a waste, and in some cases, can cause toxicity.

Give supplements time to work. Natural supplements of any kind take time to show their effectiveness. They are not like pharmaceutical drugs, which work quickly. In some cases, it may take two weeks and up to a month for a supplement to build up to its therapeutic level.

ALWAYS discuss the supplements you are taking with your physician. You want to use supplements to enhance, and never to block or counteract, the effectiveness of any other treatments you are undergoing under a physician's care. The presence of a substance in your blood also needs to be known, and factored in to the results of blood tests.

Even if your physician isn't a believer in natural cancer-resistance therapies, there is no benefit and can actually be harm in keeping secrets from your doctor. *Don't do it.*

7

Living in Balance

S ome who practice natural medicine make this statement: "A cancer diagnosis is a sign that your life is out of balance." There is a truth to explore in those words for those of us interested in cancer resistance. Nonetheless, being able to understand and use the wisdom they contain can depend on some very personal factors.

For instance, depending upon your mood or temperament, and whether you carry a fundamental guilt, you can hear this statement—"cancer is a signal that your life is out of balance"—as a criticism or condemnation. Your translation of those words will be: "If I'd just been living in balance, this wouldn't have happened to me. Look what I've brought upon myself. I'm not sure *what* I did wrong, but somehow this is my fault."

If you think like this, you're likely to tack on this corollary: "And if I just figure out how to get my life in balance again, my cancer will disappear. I'll be cured."

This is what happens when you live on the frosty spiritual ground of "permaguilt." You'll imagine that you and you alone are responsible for preventing or curing an incursion of cancer. And in doing so you'll take on an unnecessary load of stress.

The fact is, even wonderfully balanced people contract cancer all the time. Other factors apart from our doing are at work on us every day. The onset of cancer is *not* "proof" that we're at fault. And even in cases where long-term negligence or abuse of our health *might* be a factor, agonizing and berating ourselves will do nothing to help us heal. Guilt and the wrenching stress it spreads through body, mind, and spirit only works against us.

If in reading these words you realize that a sense of guilt is the deep ground on which your spirit walks on pained feet…if feeling at fault is fundamental to the way you think…if guilt drives you to do much of what you do…it's time to detox yourself of that poison. Because guilt—when left unchecked—always spreads. It moves out from your spirit where it's lodged, negatively affecting your mind and body…moving out beyond you in your words and actions (and nonactions) until it has tainted your whole approach to life and living, work and play, and your relationships with other people and with God.

Dealing with guilt, for many of us, is the first step in moving toward balance…and toward health and wholeness as well.

The Wisdom of a Balanced Life

There *is* wisdom in living a balanced life, and it's this: Balanced living undeniably promotes overall health and well-being, and it makes you more resilient and able to recover even from major illnesses. Once again, getting your life in balance is not a metaphysical "magic bullet"—a sure preventative or cure for cancer. But some important health benefits come when you make a commitment to balanced living. These benefits include:

→ the development of self-care habits (vs. self-neglect) that support overall health;

→ a keener awareness about the state of our body, mind, and spirit that helps us spot when something is wrong (vs. missing problems) and that allows us to respond by checking out potential health problems and treating them sooner;

→ a keener awareness of conflicts and stresses (vs. ignoring them) that allows us to resolve stresses quickly, triggering the deep-relaxation response that boosts the whole immune system.

But what does it mean to live in balance? How do you restore balance when you're living out of order or in tension?

To make this practical and useful, we're going to look at some of the most common ways we all tend to live out of balance. You should approach the following section in the spirit of healthy self-examination, not an inquisition. It will help you to identify specific aspects of your life where imbalance exists. Where there is imbalance, there is always stress in some measure. And stress wears us down physically, mentally, or spiritually, eroding our health.

To this point, we've looked at specific strategies to help boost resilience in various aspects of your life. Discovering imbalances will help you correct the aspects of your life that are weakening your overall health and leaving you susceptible to the ravages of a major illness. Most of all, it will help give you a bigger picture of your life. It will help you see the greater work you can do—the work of really living, regardless of the physical state you find yourself in at any given moment.

Maintaining Balance—A Self-Examination

As you use this self-examination, keep this important idea in mind:

Balance is not something we achieve once and for all—like earning a college degree. Rather, we learn how to keep balance in our lives, similar to the way we learn the simple art of riding a bike.

As it is when riding a bike, keeping balance in our lives requires us to make constant small adjustments—compensating for a big bump here, shifting our emphasis over there. If this sounds like a bit of work, it is. But only at first. When we first learn how to ride, we have to concentrate fairly carefully. We have to become mindful of problems and imbalances in order to correct and not ignore them. But eventually the adjustments we must make to stay balanced become second nature. As it is with riding a bike, so it is with life.

The good news is, if we make these efforts we develop a kind of mastery in our lives and our well-being. Personally, I believe this is what the New Testament writer meant, in part, when he spoke of the spiritual gift of "self-control." Self-control comes, at least in this natural sense, from developing a sort of "control center"—a quiet, objective core-self…one that knows how to recognize the effects of poor choices and also how to make better, healthier choices.

Whether or not you see personal balance as a spiritual matter, or merely as an aid to good health and disease resistance, the fact remains: The more we maintain our balance, the less stress we carry.

And the less stress we carry, the stronger our overall health and our ability to resist illness and disease will be.

What follows are questions to help you get some idea of the balance you're achieving right now in various aspects of your life. The questions posed under each heading are not exhaustive by any means. But these questions will help raise key issues and other important questions for you. This is purposeful, because good questions start us on good quests…and life isn't much if it's not a quest for the better.

Specifically, use these questions to help you recognize places in your life where imbalances are stressing and wearing you down, compromising your health and ability to recover from illness.

And, of course, take time to decide how you can correct the imbalances you discover.

Your Physical Balance

Maintaining physical balance, on the simplest level, means giving our bodies what they need to function at their best. Many of us have specific health issues that must also be taken into consideration. But we create a fundamental physical well-being when we balance:

Self-Care…"Body Image." One component of physical well-being has to do with taking care of ourselves, (taking responsibility for our appearance and our health). If we're neglectful, or give other people too much authority to make physical healthcare decisions for us, we're giving away power and responsibility—and life doesn't work as well.

Balance in this area of living also has another component—that's the way we relate to our bodies…our "body image." If we're displeased or embarrassed about some part of our body or appearance (and who isn't?), we may tend to ignore and neglect that part of ourselves.

- *Do I take care of my physical body?* Or do I ignore exercise and dietary needs? Do I let dental care slip? Do I have regular physical checkups? Do I use that old excuse, "I just don't like going to the doctor" to cover the real reasons I'm lax about healthcare needs?

- *Do I have a problem with my body?* Or am I frustrated because of some impairment? Do I reject something about the way I look? Do I ignore grooming and bathing? Do I live in opposition to my own physical being in some way...or am I committed to doing the best I can with what I have? What's my relationship to my physical person?

Work...Rest. Our body needs to work—that is, our muscles need exercise to work them out. Sitting at a desk in front of a computer, or driving a car all day, or even chasing kids around all day—however fatiguing—is *not* a workout. (Here's me, ducking the flying bricks.)

Our body also needs rest. Given the fact that experts say the vast majority of adults are sleep deprived, it's possible the most important adjustment you can make right now is to be in bed asleep by 10:00. For those who approach life as a spiritual mission, I will quote a friend who is a monk: "It's hard for the Spirit to work when you're tired and miserable."

- *Do you really get decent physical workouts?* Or do I feel fatigued from storing stress in my muscles all day and convince myself I'm too tired for even a brief (30-minute) workout? Do I let illness or impairment keep me from doing basic workouts (stretching, deep breathing, low-impact aerobics)?

- *Do I get enough sleep and rest?* Or do I push myself to the brink and then "crash"? Do I live in a tired fog and tell myself I can't afford to rest? What's my relationship to the way I expend energy...and restore it?

Mindful Eating...Celebrating. The body does not work right without proper fuel and nutrition. We need to eat mindfully—that is, knowing what we specifically need to eat to maintain our health and proper weight. Otherwise we're just eating without any relationship between what we put in our mouths and our actual physical needs.

On the other side, food has always been part of celebrating life. Some of us have become so bound by diet and weight and self-image needs that food has become an enemy. *Food is not our enemy.* The shallowness of people who would reject us based on our appearance is the issue. Specific illnesses or food allergies is the issue. Celebrating life by enjoying great food can make us grateful for the gift of life.

- *Do I pay attention to my dietary and exercise needs? Do I regularly make adjustments to these regimens, as needed?* Or do I more or less ignore good dietary and exercise information and "do my own thing"? Do I binge on diet and exercise when I need to lose weight—and wind up yo-yoing?

- *Do I misuse food, by overeating a lot or by seeing food as an enemy? Do I see it as a way to celebrate life on special occasions?* What is my relationship with food...and with living?

Your Mind

In the same way our body can benefit from right diet, exercise, and natural tonics...our minds can benefit from what we put into them, how we use them, and mental "tonics." Mental well-being comes from reaching balances, like these:

Mind-Feeding...and Mind "Candy." Our mind needs healthy challenges. It needs questions and new ideas to help it stretch. It needs new ways of viewing the world to keep it flexible. It needs to hear from greater minds to become strong.

Our mind also needs "lighter fare" to keep it vibrant and youthful. It needs humor. Wonder. Play.

- *Do I give my mind the healthy challenges it needs to stretch, stay flexible, and be strong? Do I keep a mental quest going by reading good books, going to seminars, seeking out new ideas?* Or do I feed it "TV Dinners"? Do I let other people do the thinking for me? Is my attitude: "My mind is made up and I have all the answers...so don't bother me with new facts or opinions"?

- *Do I "lighten up" my mental atmosphere by enjoying good humor and entertainment?* Or is my "mind candy" really just garbage?

Examining Our Thoughts...Allowing Unchallenged New Ideas.
Examining our thoughts leads us to the mental strength we know as
conviction. And conviction gives us a solid stance from which to
speak and act.

We also need to allow ourselves to explore new ideas unchallenged—that is, without knuckling in to the interior voices that say,
"I shouldn't think this way," or "I'm not intelligent enough to think
this through," or "I don't want to think about this—because it challenges a conclusion I thought I'd reached."

In short, we encourage mental resilience by balancing times
when we examine our own thoughts to see if they hold up to
reality...with times for free thought and speculation.

- *Do I take time to examine my thoughts to see if they're logi-
  cally sound—that is, connected to reality? After I think things
  through, do I stand by my conclusions?* Or do I let emotion
  wipe out reason? Am I afraid to examine my thoughts
  because they might not be well founded after all? Do I let
  others undermine my thoughts and convictions just because
  they wear some badge of authority?

- *Do I allow myself time to escape censoring inner voices and free
  think about new possibilities and solutions and better answers
  to old questions?*

Intense Thinking...Forward-moving Thinking. Intense thinking
is like "going for the burn" in mental-workout terms. Thinking
deeply *into* an issue gives us a strong base of confidence from which
to speak and act.

Note: If you're plagued by obsessive thinking—by thoughts that
repeat over and over—it may be a sign of Obsessive-Compulsive
Disorder or another mental/emotional problem. I encourage you
to seek help from a knowledgeable professional.

We need more than a base for thinking, or we'll tend to be stuck
doing things the same way over and over. We can also reject new
ideas and new people who are not "like-minded," and thus become
isolated. We need progressive thoughts, from new sources, to help us
learn more and more about the world around us and the people
who live in it.

- *Do I think things through?* Or do I act and react mostly without thinking? Do I tell myself, "I'm not very smart"? Am I intimidated, or jealous, of "brainy" people? Do I excuse myself in some other way from mental exercise?

- *Do I listen to new ideas and other people's view?* Or am I threatened by different perspectives? Do I get nervous when someone voices a view different from mine—so that I stop listening and just prepare a forceful rebuttal? Am I really *so* weak that I can't listen…and learn *something?*

Your Emotions

The mind is not just logical thought. Inside our head, logical thoughts mix with the flow of feelings that bubble up from those deeper places inside us. Emotions can be a powerful force for good or ill. If we ignore or "stuff" emotions, they can eventually sneak up on us as physical, mental, or spiritual ailments. In the range of important emotional needs, here are a few of the foundational ones where balance is important to overall health.

Expressed Emotion…Directed Emotion. Emotions are raw energy.

We need to express emotions—especially the negative ones—rather than let their energy eat at us from within.

On the other hand, one thing that makes us human—not mention in possession of a healthy self—is our ability to decide what to do with the raw energy of our feelings. What we need is a balance of "meeting" and knowing our own emotions…and then choosing how to use their energy in healthy ways.

Recent thinking in some parts of the therapeutic community says it's best to "just let it all out." Other forces in our culture tell us emotions are dangerous, shameful, or they make us "weak." Is there any question we need help finding emotional balance?

On one hand, we're out of balance if we believe there is nothing we can do to resolve raw feelings like grief, anger, or fear. We remain stuck in the past and fail to get on with the rest of living. On the other hand, it's really *not* in our best interest always to act on an emotional impulse. People who are emotionally reactive often waste their energy on emotional outbursts.

What about working out a healthy new balance in our lives by directing our energies into changing unhealthy, unhappy situations and resolving problems?

- *Do I express my emotions? Do I even know what I feel?* Or do I ignore emotions to the point where I minimize them out of existence? Do I belittle myself when I feel sad, angry, or fearful?

- *Do I direct my emotional energies into making healthy, real changes?* Or do I blow off steam and fail to follow through by making healthy changes? Do I excuse myself from working for change, saying, "It's useless," or "It doesn't matter"?

Dependence…Independence…Cooperation. Healthy relationships help to give us emotional well-being. Learning how and when to rely on others…how and when to rely on ourselves…and when to be interdependent—these emotional skills take time to balance.

- *Do I depend on other people when I need to? Do I know my limitations and needs?* Or am I invested in hiding my needs and limitations? Am I afraid to ask for help because people will look down on me…or because I don't think I can handle the disappointment if they fail to come through? Do I know how to ask for what I need—or do I think people who love me should just *know* what I need?

- *Do I operate independently whenever, wherever the need to do so arises?* Or am I overly dependent on other people for some… most…all…of my needs? Do I feel incapable of handling some aspect of life on my own, even temporarily? Do I feel anxious or panicky, at the thought of shouldering some emotional responsibility by myself?

- *Do I know how to cooperate…and be interdependent…doing some things for you and letting you do some things for me?* Or do I have to be in charge of the whole show? Do I have to be right? Do I micromanage people and projects…until I drive them away?

Light Relationships…Deep Relationships. Life is richer, and we tend to be healthier, when we enjoy a range of relationships.

We need some relationships, with people who are just fun, "social" contacts who share some surface interest with us—be it sport fishing, or chess, or the play-offs on TV, or the opera. We don't need deep attachments to everyone we know.

On the other hand, we also need *some* deeper relationships, with people who know our history, our strengths, and our weaknesses. We need people who know us well and like us anyway—and who are loyal and brave enough to stand up to us when they see we're not acting in our own best interest. This can include standing up to us when we're not making the best health decisions.

- *Do I have light friendships that help me relax and enjoy living?* Or do I tell myself I'm too busy with work, family, and other obligations to have a good time? Do I experience a flatness and lack of interest toward life and fun? Does every relationship have to have some kind of business—or spiritual or other "agenda" to be of importance to me?

- *Do I have deeper friendships, with a shared history and loyalties to hold us together?* Or do I keep aspects of myself hidden and secret, leaving me feeling isolated? Do I resist deeper relationships because I've been betrayed or abandoned in the past, and I don't want to be at risk again? Do I know how to let supportive and "safe" people *in* to these more personal areas of my life…and how to keep *out* the ones who only criticize and condemn?

Your Spirit

Spirit is that foundational level of our being created by our ideals and beliefs. It's where our mind and emotions check in to see if "all's right" or "something's wrong" with the world we are particularly living in. If we're willing to be honest and grow to maturity, it's where we check in to see if the problem we sense is *really* with the world…or if it's with us.

An imbalance in the spirit pitches our whole life into upheaval. If we ignore what our spirit is saying, we do so at our own peril. In the end, the codes by which we gauge the rightness of things *will* win out. They are supposed to. We each need a spiritual compass to navigate by.

Spiritual balance comes as we pay attention to:

Interior Growth...Interior Rest. Growth in spirit comes from having our values, ideals, and beliefs tested. We ask, we seek, we knock...we grow.

Spiritual rest comes from knowing that, even when life's greatest challenges strike, we are not abandoned and doomed but that God is at work on our behalf. Inner rest comes from laying aside our quests and questions and learning to rest in the hands of a God who upholds all things...even when life is chaotic and painful.

- *Do I test my ideals, values, and beliefs against reality? If they clash, do I allow myself to stretch and grow to find a more accurate approach to life?* Or am I rigidly dogmatic? Do I openly or secretly judge people, and avoid them or cut them out of my "fellowship"?

- *Do I have a quiet core—a sanctuary of the spirit—where I can go to, to find nurture and strength in God?* Or do I live at a busy, even hectic pace, giving no attention to cultivating my spirit? Does being alone and quiet make me feel anxious? Bored? Empty? Fearful?

Community...Solitude. We come to know ourselves and our place in the world when we interact with other people—especially people who are committed to spiritual causes...be it prayer, social service, or social justice. When we're in need we find support in communities.

As well, we also come to know ourselves by stepping apart and recognizing our differences and disagreements. We find personal strength in letting our beliefs carry us through tough times.

Spiritual balance comes by identifying with a group—but not being swallowed by it. It also comes from learning to speak up about blindness and weakness in the community we're part of.

- *Am I connected to a group by shared beliefs or commitments?* Or do I keep my distance from spiritual communities? Do I feel they're unnecessary, or hypocritical? Am I a "member" of a community—but feel alone in a crowd, or anonymous, there?

- *Can I be strong apart from my spiritual community? Are my ideals, values, and beliefs* really *mine?* Or am I afraid to test what I believe out on my own? Has experience given me insight or wisdom…or a new opinion…my spiritual community needs to hear?

Legacy…Immediate Demands. Our ideals, values, and beliefs express themselves in the goals we give our time, energy, and money to achieve.

Working for a legacy means to work for goals that are beyond our own personal needs. We learn to invest ourselves for the benefit of others—whether that means an investment of time, energy, or finances.

Working for our personal needs is also essential, though, for spiritual balance. We are not angels yet, and we live healthier when we keep money and possessions in their proper place…*after* spiritual values…but still important in this very real world.

- *Do I have commitments to "missions" that will benefit others? Am I building a legacy of a better world and changed lives?* Or am I spending my time, energy, and money just on myself, on fun, or on possessions?

- *Am I overcommitted to "helping others" and stinting on my own, or my family's immediate needs?* Do I need to take care of real immediate needs, for the sake of my own well-being and comfort…or that of my family?

Your Vital Energies

There is a sense in which we need to look at our own vital energies apart from physical exercise, mental effort, or the effort we put into spiritual activities. Vitality rises when we're living passionately…and ebbs when we are not. In that sense, it can be a barometer of our resilience to illness and ability to recover when disease strikes.

Stepping back and looking at our own level of vitality—how much we have, and how we use it—can often give us a bigger view of our lives…and tell us a lot about whether or not we're living in or out of balance.

"Your" Work … "Your" Recreation. We feel vitalized by working at a job that we care about. We are revitalized by play that gives us joy and forgetfulness of our duties and cares.

- *Am I passionate about my work? Do I even like my work?* Or am I just working for a paycheck? Do I have future goals…giving my energies to achieve a vision I have for myself and my life?

- *Do I have a passion outside of work?* Or is my life a rutted cowpath of work, duties, obligations, time spent meeting other people's concerns, needs, or demands? Do I even know what would make me happy and revitalized again?

Commitment to Yourself…Commitment to Others…Commitment to God. Committing time and energy into ourselves, into others, and into our relationship with God gives life a healthy balance. *Commitment* is the operative word here.

A commitment to ourselves means we do not give up on ourselves. We love and care for ourselves—body, mind, and spirit. We do what is best for our balance and well-being.

A commitment to others means we do not give up on family and friends. We cannot direct their lives…but we do not abandon them. We do what we can for their good.

A commitment to God means we do not give up on pressing into the wonder…or the mysteries of God's presence and work in our lives.

- *Do I have a commitment to care for my body, mind, and spirit?* Or do I spend all my energies maintaining other people's needs? Do I give more attention to my work or possessions than to my own physical, mental, or spiritual well-being?

- *Do I have a commitment to caring for friends?* Or do I neglect building true relationships, leaving myself without loyal companions or support when I'm in need?

- *Do I have a commitment to growing in a relationship with God?* Or am I blind to the wonder and reality of God? Do I have God "all figured out," so I am not challenged by mysteries about God's ways? Am I angry or fearful of letting my thoughts, feelings, or true opinions be known to God?

The Art of Living

To be really alive is an art. It takes effort to balance all the aspects of our life until we're experiencing vitality and overall well-being. This great vitality is also one of the most potent means of resisting sickness and disease.

My hope is that the ideas we've explored in this book will continue to help you maintain healthy balances in your life. And that it will benefit you greatly in your efforts to resist cancer.

The New Nature Institute

The New Nature Institute was founded in 1999 for the purpose of exploring the connection between personal health and wellness and spirituality, with the Hebrew-Christian tradition as its spiritual foundation.

Drawing upon this tradition, the Institute supports the belief that humankind is created in the image of God. We are each body, mind, and spirit and so intricately connected that each aspect of our being affects the other. If one aspect suffers, our whole being suffers; if all aspects are being supported, we will enjoy a greater sense of well-being.

For this reason, the Institute engages in ongoing research in order to provide up-to-date information that supports a "whole-person" approach to wellness. Most especially, research is focused on the natural approaches to wellness that supports health and vitality in the body, the mind, and the spirit.

Healthy Body, Healthy Soul is a series of books intended to complement treatment plans provided by healthcare professionals. They are not meant to be used in place of professional consultations and/or treatment plans.

Along with creating written materials, the New Nature Institute also presents seminars, workshops, and retreats on a range of topics relating to spirituality and wellness. These can be tailored for corporate, spiritual community, or general community settings.

For information contact:
The New Nature Institute
Attn: David Hazard
P.O. Box 568
Round Hill, Virginia 20142
(540) 338-7032
Exangelos@ aol.com